Rochester History

FALL 2024

Rochester History

A publication of the Rochester Public Library
in partnership with Rochester Institute of Technology

Volume 82, Issue 1

Contents

DIRECTOR'S CORNER

This issue of *Rochester History* illuminates a period of time in our history where the right of women to control their own bodies became paramount. Elizabeth Carr provides a startling and informative investigation into the early work of community members to provide safe and affordable birth control to women who needed it. One hundred years later, women are still advocating for their rights, although clearly there have been significant advances in health-care options since the era Carr discusses. This factual look at how Rochester's first birth control clinic began and evolved through the years offers a stark view into the struggle of women to manage their motherhood. Birth control remains a hot-button issue in the twenty-first century, and this look at its early twentieth-century scope is remarkable. ■

Patricia Uttaro
Director, Rochester Public Library & Monroe County Library System

Dear reader,

We are pleased to welcome you to our Fall 2024 issue.

In an election-year news cycle that has been deeply shaped by post-Dobbs politics, we are especially fortunate to provide our readers with a deep dive into the history of women's reproductive rights in Rochester. In this issue's main feature, Elizabeth Carr invites us all to consider "Birth Control on a Local Level: The Monroe County Birth Control League, 1934–1945." As Carr makes clear, there has never been a time, in our nation's history or in our local history, when these very personal matters were not politically charged.

We offer a review essay on another weighty political matter: racial segregation in schools and in cities. Richard D. Deverell brings two books together in his review of Justin Murphy's *Your Children Are Very Greatly in Danger*, which focuses on racial segregation in the Rochester school system, and father-daughter writing team Richard and Leah Rothstein's *Just Action*, which confronts practices of racial segregation in city planning.

Meanwhile, in another review, Erik Seeman delves into Rochester's religious past with his consideration of Spencer W. McBride and Jennifer Hull Dorsey's *New York's Burned-Over District: A Documentary History*.

But this will not be your only chance to explore Rochester's religious history in this issue! We are pleased to offer a new feature to you, "Teaching the ROC." If you have ever wondered what the view of the classroom is like from behind the podium, Teaching the ROC will take you there. In the inaugural edition of this feature, Daniel J. Gorman Jr. takes you on a backstage tour of one of his college classes. Join him in HIST 326: Digital History as he guides students on an intellectual adventure called "The Hill Cumorah Legacy Project: Capturing Rochester's Latter-Day Saint History."

Can't get enough pedagogy? Don't worry—there's more! Our digital edition provides bonus content. You can follow the project along, from conception to completion, in an extended version of Teaching the ROC. We hope to inspire both learners and teachers alike with this feature.

Finally, ROC Artifact returns. In this edition, Cynthia Van Ness brings us an unusual item to consider: a wallpaper sample from the Hotel Seneca. If you had been a guest at the downtown hotel in 1908, this is the wallpaper that would have greeted you as you moved through the hotel's corridors. What you probably would not have known is that the designer behind the paper was Moses Shongo, a member of the Seneca Nation. Turn to the ROC Artifact to see the sample and to learn more about Shongo himself. Enjoy! ■

Christine L. Ridarsky and Rebecca Edwards
Editors

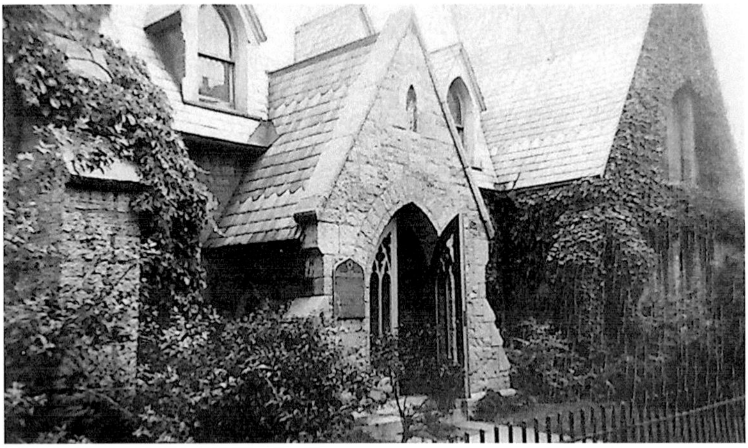

Owned by the First Unitarian Church, the basement of the Gannett House was the Rochester Clinic's first home. *Gannett House, Series IX, Folder 20, Unitarian Church, Rochester, New York papers, D.54, Rare Books, Special Collections, & Preservation, River Campus Libraries, University of Rochester.*

Birth Control on a Local Level: The Monroe County Birth Control League, 1934–1945

by Elizabeth Carr

In the twenty-first century, the name Planned Parenthood brings to mind *Roe v. Wade*, debates over abortion, and a polarizing national organization. It's easy to assume Planned Parenthood has always operated under these conditions, but its modern iteration is vastly different from the birth control clinics of the early to mid-twentieth century. Long before abortion access was part of a national conversation, the earliest birth control clinics were locally founded, funded, and operated and were designed to provide lower-income women with access to family planning services and devices.[1] History suggests that such facilities operated uniformly and that a focus on preventing certain individuals from having children and on forced or coerced birth control, along with widespread public opposition to birth control practices, were national trends in this era. However, as Rochester's first birth control clinic demonstrates, local and regional variances existed. Viewing early birth control clinics through a local lens helps bring such discrepancies into focus, complicating—yet clarifying—the national picture.

Rochester's first birth control clinic opened on February 21, 1934.[2] Like many early American clinics, it provided working-class women with family planning services and birth control devices. And like many clinics, it also faced opposition from religious authorities. Yet the clientele it served and the methods

Elizabeth Carr is a PhD candidate in history at the University of Rochester, with an emphasis on nineteenth- and twentieth-century US history. Her research focuses on the intersection of museums, public history, and digital technology and how they can enhance people's engagement with the past.

it prescribed were different from those commonly accepted as typical across the United States during this period. In looking at Rochester clinic records, personal reflections from its founders, data about patients and services, and reading materials the clinic published, one sees certain patterns emerge.[3] Namely, it becomes clear that Rochester was unique in the devices it prescribed and the predominantly Catholic clientele it served, though the economic status of its patrons mirrored the demographics of women who sought resources from similar clinics across the country. The clinic's records also help elucidate the environment in which the clinic was founded and developed—that of a mid-sized city in the midst of the Great Depression, with a specific population demographic and class structure.[4]

On a more granular level, these records provide insights into the people who founded and staffed the clinic during its nascent years. Until at least the mid-1940s, the Monroe County Birth Control League was not affiliated with the umbrella organization of Planned Parenthood, meaning that the impetus for its establishment and its early operations were tied to members of the local Rochester community.[5] Generally speaking, the founders were upper-class women who came from considerable wealth. As members of Rochester's high society, their travels and multiple club activities were regularly reported on in the local newspapers. They were married to men who held high-ranking jobs, but they rarely had careers of their own, giving them the time and resources to devote to the clinic and a host of other clubs. Though they took part in several organizations, their participation in the clinic was seemingly not disingenuous. Many founders demonstrated a vested interest in, and dedication to, the clinic's success even years after their involvement. Marjorie Harris Reynolds, for example, was elected the Monroe County Birth Control League's treasurer in 1935; her 1989 obituary asked for donations to be made to Rochester's Planned Parenthood clinic in lieu of flowers.[6] For some founders, such philanthropic work seemed to be connected to part of a larger desire to specifically advocate for women. Marcia Ellingson, an early clinic board member and the wife of former Rochester Institute of Technology president Mark Ellingson, noted in her 1973 reminiscences: "After my marriage in 1934 there were several easy steps from my membership on the Board of the League of Women Voters to acceptance of the invitation to the Board of Planned Parenthood in 1939."[7] The reflections of these women are crucial to understanding how the clinic functioned during its early days and the ways in which Rochester mirrored or diverged from national trends regarding contraception.

Who Ran the Clinic?

Ruth H. Backus (née Haven) was the executive director of the Monroe County Birth Control League from 1934 to 1954. Like many of the women involved with the clinic, Backus was a wealthy member of Rochester society. Her husband, Sidney Backus, was an attorney and later served as Webster town supervisor. They were both members of numerous social organizations in Rochester, such as the American Red Cross, the Home Bureau, and the Girl Scouts.[1] Backus differed from a number of her colleagues in that she held a degree in liberal arts from Wellesley College and had worked as a social worker at Genesee Hospital prior to her taking the job at the clinic. Her formal training suggests that her involvement with the clinic was in a more professional capacity than that of many of the volunteers, and it undoubtedly helped prepare her for her duties as director.

Margaret "Miggie" Baum (née Hays) was a founding member of the Monroe County Birth Control League and a lifelong advocate for birth control and other philanthropic causes. She was born in Rochester and received a degree in English from Smith College. Her husband, Morton Baum, was the president of Hickey-Freeman Co. from 1959 until his death in 1963. Baum was a member of the Red Cross, worked with societies that promoted assisted suicide, and was involved in Planned Parenthood at the local, state, and federal levels for more than fifty years.[2]

Ruth Briggs (née Curtis) was a member of the clinic's board of directors in the 1940s and likely a volunteer during the 1930s. She was a Rochester native whose husband, Theodore Briggs, briefly served as Rochester city manager. Briggs was a homemaker who was deeply involved with a number of local organizations, including the Girl Scouts Council and Women's Overseas Service League. She also served as a nurse's aide in France during World War I and as a Captain of the Red Cross Motor Corps in World War II.[3]

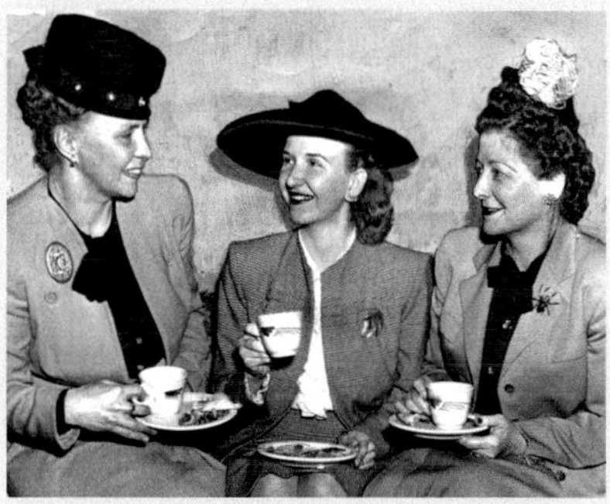

Marcia Ellingson, seated on the left, was the wife of RIT President Mark Ellingson, as well as a board member of the birth control clinic and one of its earliest volunteers. In this 1946 image, she sits with two other members of the RIT Women's Club, another charitable group she founded. *RIT Women's Club Records (RIT Archives.0005).*

Marcia Ellingson (née Randall) was the daughter of John Randall, the president of Rochester Institute of Technology from 1922 to 1936, and married Mark Ellingson, who served as RIT's president from 1936 to 1969. She was active in a number of philanthropic endeavors in Rochester, most notably the birth control clinic where she was a board member, but she was also involved with the Monroe County League of Women Voters and a number of organizations concerned with improving conditions for women faculty and students at RIT. She received the Susan B. Anthony Civic Award in 1967 for her contributions to Rochester's civic life and was a lifelong advocate for women's rights and sexual education.[4]

Florence King (née Hoerner) was a founding member of the Rochester clinic and was deeply involved with its operations for many years. Her husband, Edmund King, was an assistant treasurer at the Eastman Kodak Company, while Florence was a homemaker and a member of numerous clubs in Rochester. Many of these organizations were religiously affiliated, with King serving as a trustee, church-school leader, board member, and delegate at Brick Presbyterian Church. However, she was also involved in secular causes such as the clinic, the Pittsford Community Library, and the Girl Scouts.[5]

Dr. Saul Moress was the son of Russian Jewish immigrants and attended the University of Rochester before receiving his medical degree from Cornell University. He lived in the city of Rochester with his wife, Rose, and their two children. The Moresses appear to have been involved in numerous social activities in the local Jewish community, with Rose appearing in plays and Saul giving public lectures and serving as the music council chairman for the Jewish Young Men's and Women's Association Symphony Orchestra. The family seemingly fared well financially but was not part of the same social circles as the clinic's volunteers.[6]

Marjorie Reynolds (née Harris) was a member of the Rochester clinic's board of trustees, as well as a member of many organizations in the Rochester area. She came from a wealthy family and was married to August Oddleifson, a broker at L.F. Rothschild & Co., during her time at the clinic. Reynolds was mentioned in the *Democrat and Chronicle* numerous times throughout the 1930s and the

Birth Control in Rochester

The Rochester clinic was established during the Great Depression, a period that had a considerable impact on attitudes toward birth control. Beginning in late 1929 and lasting through the 1930s, the Great Depression was a profound economic recession that affected Americans of all backgrounds and income levels. These difficult circumstances led to a shift in general attitudes toward contraception, with many starting to favor birth control and family planning due to the financial strains a child could put on a hard-pressed family. As historian Rickie Solinger states in *Pregnancy and Power: A Short History of Reproductive*

1950s, with her name being connected with the Rochester Children's Nursery, the Chatterbox Club, and the Monroe County Defense Savings Committee, among other local institutions. She appears to have not held a career and mostly devoted her time to homemaking and volunteer efforts.[7]

1 "Obituary: Ruth Backus, birth control activist," *Democrat and Chronicle*, February 15, 1988; "Red Cross Meet Draws 23 of City," *Democrat and Chronicle*, May 23, 1957; "Overnight Hike of Troop 21," *Democrat and Chronicle*, June 14, 1924.

2 Deborah Fineblum Raub, "Miggie Baum starts things," *Democrat and Chronicle*, July 13, 1986, 6D; Andy Smith, "Margaret Baum, at our service," *Democrat and Chronicle*, August 16, 1982, 1C.

3 "Ruth Curtis Briggs," *The Stuart News*, May 27, 1987; Untitled, *Democrat and Chronicle*, January 2, 1930; Untitled, *Democrat and Chronicle*, October 3, 1935; "Theodore C. Briggs dies at 92, former head of Lawyers Co-op," *Democrat and Chronicle*, December 19, 1984.

4 M. Kathleen Wagner, "Marcia Ellingson, 82; RIT 'First lady' women's activist," *Democrat and Chronicle*, April 15, 1993; "Mrs. Ellingson Honored," *Democrat and Chronicle*, April 27, 1967.

5 "Florence King, founder of city Planned Parenthood," *Democrat and Chronicle*, February 2, 1982.

6 "Moress, Saul MD," *Democrat and Chronicle*, May 12, 1984; "JY Symphony Lists Season Opening," *Democrat and Chronicle*, December 11, 1949; "Mrs. Saul Moress/Mrs. Lucille Michel," *Democrat and Chronicle*, January 29, 1939; "Speaker Announced for JYM-WA Forum," *Democrat and Chronicle*, March 12, 1939; "Former U.R. Men Hospital Internes," *Democrat and Chronicle*, July 30, 1927; US Census Bureau, *Fifteenth Census of the United States: 1930*, Rochester, NY, Block No. 349, 236.

7 "August G. Oddleifson, Broker, Succumbs," *Democrat and Chronicle*, October 21, 1936; "What Women Will be [*sic*] Doing This Week," *Democrat and Chronicle*, February 21, 1965; "Brighton Opens New Stamp Outlets," *Democrat and Chronicle*, April 2, 1942; "Nursery Picks Mrs. Gleason," *Democrat and Chronicle*, April 30, 1937; "Mrs. Harris Leaves $751,057 to Children," *Democrat and Chronicle*, December 23, 1967.

Politics in America, "in this context of economic insecurity and reproductive shame and danger, many women believed that no matter what the law said, or what the church said, or what the government said was legal or illegal, birth control and abortion were basic and daily needs."[8] Additionally, the activism of groups such as Margaret Sanger's American Birth Control League, which existed from 1921 to 1938, helped birth control promotion spread across the country at a rapid pace.[9] The combination of dire economic circumstances and widespread promotion culminated in large swaths of the population accepting the use of birth control practices and implementing them into their own lives.

This shift in attitudes, however, did not mean that contraception access was equitable during the 1930s. Although the Depression hurt all social classes, some were hurt more than others. This certainly held true with respect to birth control. As Solinger points out in her work, middle- and upper-class Depression-era Americans had the means to seek out private physicians, illegal abortions, contraceptives, and information or advice.[10] Linda Gordon echoes these sentiments in *The Moral Property of Women,* stating that "although contraception became widespread in the 1930s, most middle-class people continued to get help from private doctors and most working-class and rural people, by contrast, did not get help at all."[11] The cost of contraceptives and doctor visits made birth control difficult for people in the lower socioeconomic classes to access, even though this group was decidedly interested in contraception. According to Andrea Tone in *Devices and Desires*, "the thousands of letters working-class Americans sent to Sanger and other birth control proponents reflect their view that contraceptives were not a prohibitively costly luxury but a commodity few working people could afford to be without."[12] All socioeconomic groups were interested in contraception, but only upper- and middle-class women were able to access it, leaving a void that was often filled by illegal or at-home means.

To help close this gap, hundreds of local organizations sprung up across the country in the 1930s. By December 1938, there were a reported 478 birth control clinics in the United States, of which just 97 were operated by public health departments.[13] The stories of locally operated clinics have not been well documented, meaning that there are few points of comparison for Rochester's facility. Two of the only available full-length studies focus on Cleveland, Ohio, and Houston, Texas. Maria Anderson's "Private choices vs. public voices: The history of Planned Parenthood in Houston," which discusses a clinic founded in 1936 with the aim of helping working-class families, will be used as a point of comparison for Rochester.[14] Houston had been spared the worst effects of the Great Depression due to the oil industry, but it still witnessed inequities tied to its strict racial and class segregation.[15] Like Rochester, the clinic was volunteer-run, with the staff consisting of a single physician, nurse, and administrator.[16] Although comparing a clinic in Western New York with one in Texas might seem like an odd choice, the lack of other options highlights the paucity of work that has considered birth control clinics at a local level compared to those covering national trends and demographics, which do not always account for regional variations within the United States.

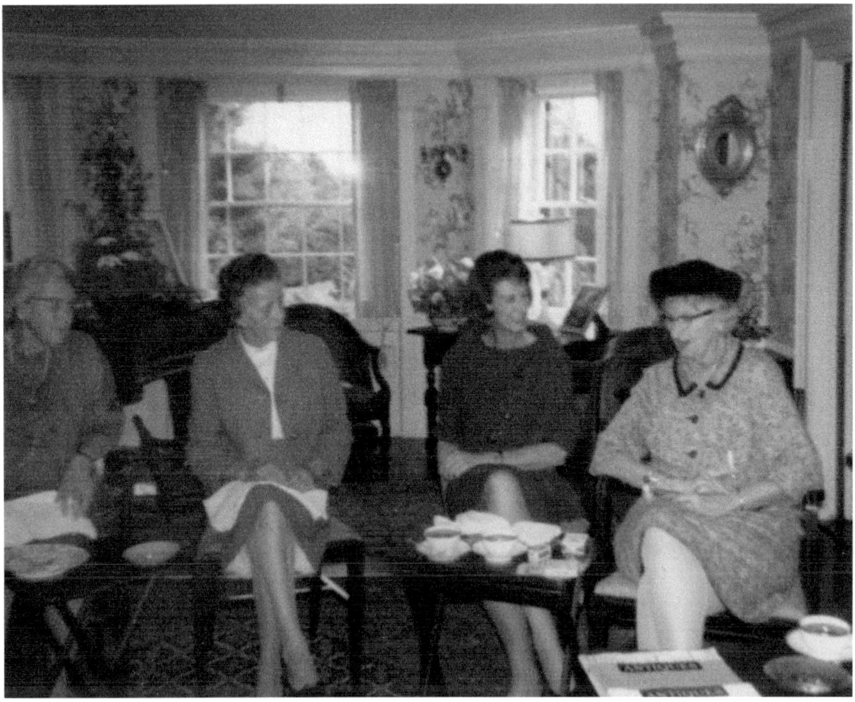

Ruth Backus, seated on the right, was the first executive director of the Rochester clinic from 1934 to 1954. Although she, like the other clinic volunteers, was from a wealthy family, Backus also had experience as a social worker prior to joining the clinic. This image was taken at a farewell party for Backus in October 1963. *Folder 3: Correspondence of Ruth Backus, Box 6, Planned Parenthood of Rochester/Syracuse Region Collection, D.325, Rare Books, Special Collections, & Preservation, River Campus Libraries, University of Rochester.*

Like many Depression-era birth control clinics across the country, Rochester's facility was established to serve working-class and underprivileged women. According to the first director of the Monroe County Birth Control League, Ruth H. Backus, interest in creating a Rochester clinic began several years before it opened. Backus wrote in "From the Cradle" that 1932 "was also the year Margaret Sanger, the leader of birth control in this country, came to Temple B'rith Kodesh. Policemen were at every door. The legality of her speech was challenged from the floor. This episode afforded much publicity, pro and con. Undoubtedly it was another factor in drawing local interest."[17] Sanger's visit seems to have elicited more positive reactions than negative; by that fall, the Monroe County Birth Control League had been established and its officers had begun working toward the goal of opening a "birth control service."[18] The early members were predominantly women from Rochester's middle and upper

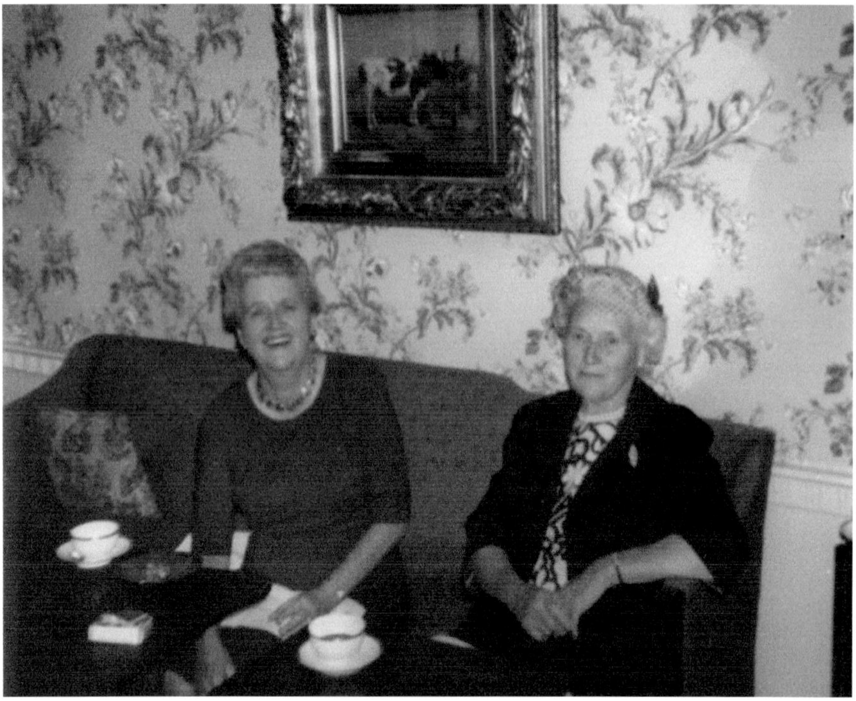
Seated on the left, Ruth Briggs was a member of the clinic's board of directors during the 1940s and was heavily involved in other philanthropic ventures in Rochester. *Folder 3: Correspondence of Ruth Backus, Box 6, Planned Parenthood of Rochester/Syracuse Region Collection, D.325, Rare Books, Special Collections, & Preservation, River Campus Libraries, University of Rochester.*

classes who felt strongly about establishing "a service for needy mothers."[19] After an initially discouraging search for a site to host the center, the First Unitarian Church offered to rent out the basement of its Gannett House, then located on Cortland Street in downtown Rochester, for $25 per week.[20] Although the Church's willingness to provide the clinic with a space was a huge step forward, the first iteration was not without its drawbacks. Former board president Ruth Briggs reminisced in 1973, "We were grateful to the Church for the years they allowed us to use it. However, there were many benefits to a place of our own. Not the least of these was the fact that we no longer had to use a pool table for examination of the Patients [*sic*]."[21] Despite its initial less-than-ideal circumstances, the clinic persevered.

The clinic officially opened in February 1934.[22] Its early staff included Backus in a part-time capacity, three physicians, and an unknown number of volunteers.[23] By the end of the year, staff had seen 245 patients. According to Miggie

Baum's 1973 reminiscences, the "first patients were women with 6 to 14 children and I recall the mother of 10 who came into our clinic, bent over, looking old and downtrodden, as she said 'I have a bottle of carbolic acid in my cellar and one more pregnancy and I'll take it.'"[24] The patient received a diaphragm and left with "her head held high." The anecdote highlights the immediate impact the clinic had on the lives and well-being of women in Rochester.

Over the course of the clinic's first year, the organization established its practices for treatment and service options. The first clinic physician, Dr. William Brown, summarized these policies in the clinic's constitution:[25]

> No patient will receive any treatment or advice whatever [*sic*] excepting contraceptive information and instruction.
>
> The contraceptive instruction will be given to those patients who have had a thorough physical (and if necessary, mental) examination, and where an honest reason, within the law, for giving that instruction is found to exist.
>
> In receiving patients, a real effort will be made to learn if that patient has a physician whom she regularly employs. If so, that physician will be consulted and if he wishes to give her this advice in his office, she will be so directed.
>
> If she has no regular physician and is able to pay a reasonable fee for this service, she will be given a list of physicians who are willing to do this work, from which list she may select the one to whom we will refer her.
>
> Patients who have no regular physician and who are manifestly unable to pay the usual charge of a private physician, will be given contraceptive instruction, if a sound reason (within the law) is found to exist.
>
> The patient, if possible, or the agency of reference, is expected to pay the cost of materials supplied in each case.[26]

The constitution included several important principles that guided the clinic in determining which patients to treat and how to treat them. First, the clinic was only responsible for providing contraceptive advice and devices. This policy differed from those of clinics operating in other parts of the country during this time, such as at the Maternal Health Center of Houston. There, "patients came in on a walk-in basis for Pap tests, to be fitted for diaphragms, to have pregnancy tests administered, and for information on child-spacing. Abortions were not performed."[27] While Houston's clinic was somewhat akin to a modern-day gynecology practice, Rochester's, by contrast, only provided contraception—without offering broader sexual-wellness services. The clinic did alert women to pregnancies if they came in for contraceptives and were found to already be pregnant, but pregnancy testing does not appear to have been one of its primary services.[28]

The difference between the Rochester and Houston clinics is due in part to the fact that New York State had banned clinics from giving contraceptive advice for non-medical reasons in the 1930s. This limitation was brought up repeatedly in reminiscences from early Monroe County Birth Control League members, who recounted operating specifically within these laws. In a 1982 letter, Ruth Backus recalled measures the clinic took: "You remember the N.Y. law permitted contraceptive [*sic*] to be prescribed by an MD to 'cure or prevent disease.' We were not allowed (no one was) to tell where contraceptives might be obtained. . . . You remember we used spacing as a medical reason."[29] The Comstock Act, a federal statute that banned sending contraceptives through the mail, was also in effect until 1938 but was not mentioned in the reminiscences of clinic volunteers or workers.[30] This suggests that state laws were of more relevance to them during this time, as these were the measures that directly affected the Rochester clinic. Such laws also ultimately contributed to regional variations among American birth control clinics of this era.

Another important tenet of the Rochester clinic's policy was to give contraceptive advice and methods only to those who were truly in need and could not obtain it from other sources. The clinic regularly turned away a significant number of women who came to them for help, most often because they were not members of the working-class population it sought to serve. During the three years for which there is full data (1939, 1940, and 1943), roughly 42 percent of refused patients were turned away for being financially ineligible for treatment.[31] Many women were also turned away in these years for not having a valid health reason to seek contraception: 41 women were refused on these grounds in 1939, followed by 38 in 1940, and 12 in 1943.[32] The 1934 constitution stated

Financial Eligibility

Year	Patients Accepted for Treatment	Patients Refused for Treatment	Number Refused for Financial Reasons	Number Refused for Health Reasons
1939	715	170	75	41
1940	598	166	62	38
1943	429	77	35	12

that these ineligible women would be sent to local private physicians to obtain contraception.[33]

Payment records further emphasize the clinic's desire to help those who were financially unable to receive contraceptives elsewhere. During the years for which such information is available, between 24 and 29 percent of patients received their services for free, while 63 to 72 percent paid between $0.01 to $1.00.[34] The clinic records do not state how the fee was determined, but given the emphasis in the constitution and other clinic documents on helping those who could not afford to visit physicians, it is safe to assume that it was based on household income or on what a patient was reasonably able to pay for the services. The clinic records for 1940 do note that 40 percent of patients were "on some form of relief, partial or wholly," and that the average wage of the employed was $19.56.[35] This data is presented without clarifying information, making it unclear if "average wage of the employed" refers to the woman, her spouse, or both. The period of time in which that wage was earned is also unknown. It should be noted, however, that according to the same document, 352 of the 598 women reported being employed full time, making it likely that this figure referred to their own wages. The records from 1943 do not include fee information, but they do state that 382 of the 429 patients seen in 1940 were "entirely self-supporting" and that another 38 were "partially supporting."[36]

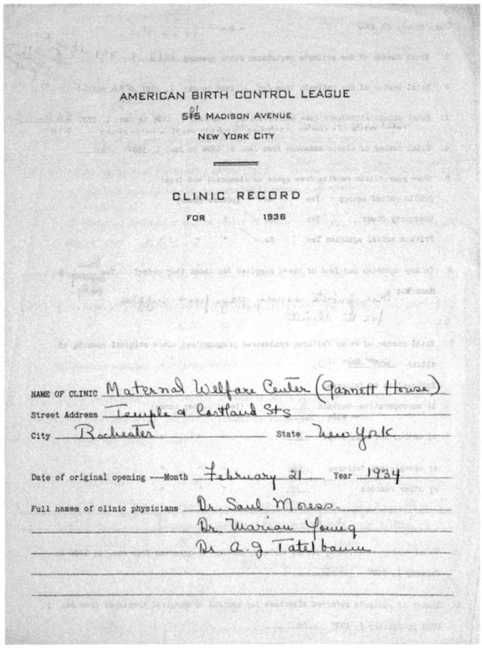
AMERICAN BIRTH CONTROL LEAGUE
515 MADISON AVENUE
NEW YORK CITY

CLINIC RECORD
FOR 1936

NAME OF CLINIC Maternal Welfare Center (Gannett House)
Street Address Temple & Cortland Sts
City Rochester State New York
Date of original opening —Month February 21 Year 1934
Full names of clinic physicians Dr. Saul Moses
Dr. Marian Young
Dr. A. J. Tatelbaum

Annual reports from the clinic report statistics such as the number of patients seen, the methods prescribed to them, and their general demographic information. Full records exist in the archive for the years 1939, 1940, and 1943. *Folder 1: Clinic Records, Box 5, Planned Parenthood of Rochester/Syracuse Region Collection, D.325, Rare Books, Special Collections, & Preservation, River Campus Libraries, University of Rochester.*

The final factor determining patient eligibility was marital status. In addition to turning away patients due to financial or health reasons, the clinic also as a rule did not treat women who were single. In 1939, thirty-four refusals were made because the women "were premaritals," while the clinic turned away

Clinic Fees

Year	Patients Accepted for Treatment	Patients Receiving Services for Free	Patients Paying $0.01 To $1.00	Other*
1939	715	209	449	57
1940	598	143	431	24

* In 1939, this number represents those paying the maximum acceptable fee. This was $2.50 for those living outside Monroe County and $2.00 for those in the county. In 1940, this is the number of patients paying $1.00 to $3.00, or $20.27 to $60.80 in 2022 dollars. *From Clinic Records, 1938, PP of Rochester/Syracuse; Clinic Records, 1939, PP of Rochester/Syracuse.*

forty-one individuals on the same grounds in 1940 and rejected thirty-five more in 1943.[37] Recalling her time spent volunteering at the clinic, Florence H. King noted in 1973, "Mind you only married, indigent women were given contraceptive advice; others were interviewed and referred to private doctors."[38] The resistance to helping unmarried women was likely influenced in part out of a desire to uphold the clinic's legitimacy to the public. As Marcia Ellingson wrote in her reminiscences, "Ruth Backus . . . directed my efforts toward treading lightly on the public resistance to words like 'birth control' and 'contraceptives.' We emphasized phrases like 'EVERY CHILD A WANTED CHILD.'"[39] In June 1939, Backus spoke at the National Conference of Social Work in Buffalo, New York, to promote this goal. In her speech, titled "The Extra-Mural Center," she stated that "the changing emphasis in a birth control program, which stresses the positive side of family planning, rather than the negative one of family limitation, is reflected in increasing use of the clinic by social workers as a preventative rather than a remedial resource."[40] In promoting birth control as a way to help families specifically, Backus was clearly making reference to the type of women birth control clinics such as Rochester's should be serving: married working-class women with low incomes and a medical need for contraception. These restrictive prerequisites suggest that the clinic may have been guided by notions of a "deserving poor" versus an "undeserving poor" and that only the former—low-income people who met moral standards dictated by members of the middle and upper classes—were worthy of aid.[41] This attitude was not uncommon among affluent philanthropists at the time. However, given the importance clinic volunteers placed on the public perception of their organization, it is difficult to determine whether they personally held such beliefs, or if they were trying to work within laws and perceptions that were already aligned with the "deserving poor" mentality.

The demographic the Monroe County Birth Control League served mirrors that of its contemporaries (for which such patient records exist). The Maternal Health Center of Houston, for example, was established to serve a similar segment of the population, focusing mainly on lower-income women who could not afford contraceptive services or did not know where to access them. As in Rochester, "all of the services and supplies were provided free, or if a woman could afford it, for fifty cents."[42] In both Houston and Rochester, local upper-class citizens founded such clinics. Patients needed to meet certain socially acceptable gender expectations as well as demonstrate financial difficulties, but these clinics helped fill a void and provided life-changing resources. In this sense, Rochester's clinic was emblematic of American birth control clinics from this period. Yet, in other significant aspects, the clinic proved atypical.

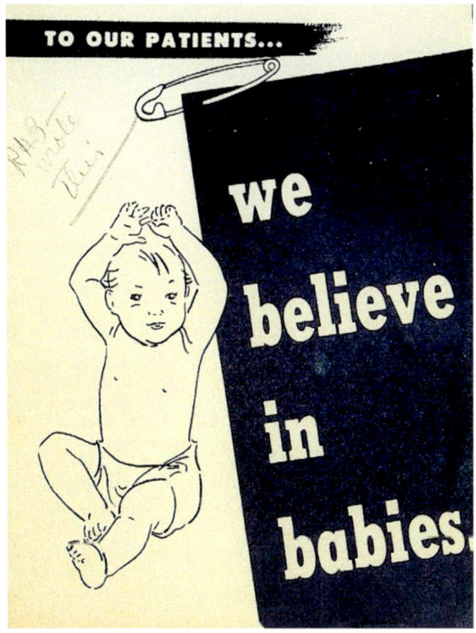

Messaging from the clinic promoted the idea of family planning over stopping women from having children. This undated pamphlet, for example, includes information such as "most of you, however, have been given advice so that you may space your children. We urge you not to wait too long for more." *Folder 2: Correspondence 1933–1937, Box 6, Planned Parenthood of Rochester/Syracuse Region Collection, D.325, Rare Books, Special Collections, & Preservation, River Campus Libraries, University of Rochester.*

Birth Control Devices

Members of the working class did not necessarily have access to the same financial or medical resources as those in the middle or upper class, and, as such, the methods they employed to prevent pregnancy often differed. The cost of medical devices, along with considerations regarding the reuse of devices, affected what women would be prescribed. Additionally, prejudiced beliefs about the intelligence level of underprivileged individuals may have influenced which devices a given doctor was willing to prescribe. In Rochester's clinic, the most recommended birth control method by far was the diaphragm used in combination with spermicidal jelly. In the 1930s and 1940s, diaphragms were one of the most reliable contraceptive methods available to women, with the caveat that they only worked well if properly fitted. Gordon indicates that in the early twentieth century, diaphragms were available for purchase at drugstores, but it was recommended that "users be fitted by a physician for reliability."[43] Tone notes in *Devices and Desires*, "Today's diaphragms are prescribed only after the cervix has been measured, a technique that enables a medical practitioner to select the best fitting size."[44] The practice of fitting diaphragms was not common when they were first introduced to consumers, but by the 1930s, doctors in Rochester fitted patients when they prescribed these methods. Reflecting on his time as the Rochester clinic's chief clinician, Dr. Saul Moress recalled that during the 1930s and 1940s, "the method of choice as [*sic*] diaphragm or jelly, or jelly, alone, if she could not be fitted with a diaphragm."[45] Ruth Backus also mentioned several times, in a 1939 article published in *The Journal of Contraception*, fitting women for diaphragms. She noted that some planned pregnancies were "not discovered until the patient comes back for a refitting," that some diaphragms were refitted by patients' own obstetricians later, and that of the thirty-three unplanned pregnancies due to device failure that the clinic saw between its opening in 1934 and the time of the article being written, eighteen of the women had "returned to the Center after childbirth for refitting."[46] Fitting patients for diaphragms was not a common practice elsewhere in the country, but in Rochester, the clinic expected to fit patients when they first visited and wanted them to return regularly for refittings. An undated clinic form titled "Patient in for Jelly" asked several questions regarding whether the birth control method the clinic prescribed was working, including, "Is diaphragm in good condition?"[47] The assumption seems to have been that most, if not all, women who received spermicidal jelly would also have received a diaphragm, and the clinic was eager to ensure they were being used as directed.

Given these repeated references from members of the Rochester clinic on the process of fitting diaphragms, it comes as no surprise that they were overwhelmingly the most popular method given to local women. During the four years for which detailed records exist, around 93 percent of new patients were prescribed a diaphragm and jelly, or, in several cases, a diaphragm and cream.[48] Other prescribed methods included condoms and jelly, jelly or cream alone, or a cervi-cap with cream or jelly. The clinic would have either given patients these devices for free or charged them according to the pay scale. Several factors contributed to the diaphragm's popularity during this period. First and foremost, properly fitted diaphragms were a reliable method of preventing pregnancy,

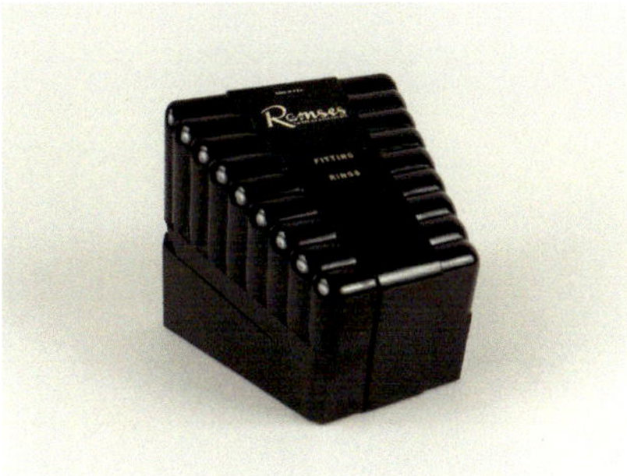

For optimal effectiveness, diaphragms came in a multitude of sizes to ensure a snug fit. These Ramses sizing rings, made circa 1930, were used by health-care providers to determine the appropriate size for patients. *Division of Medicine and Science, National Museum of American History, Smithsonian Institution.*

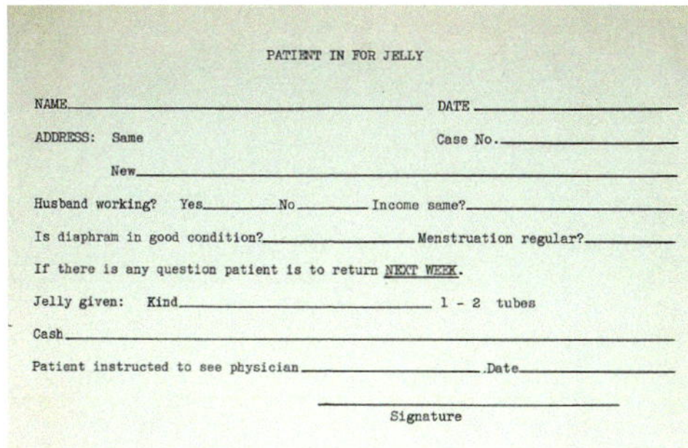

PATIENT IN FOR JELLY

NAME ____ DATE ____

ADDRESS: Same Case No. ____

New ____

Husband working? Yes ____ No ____ Income same? ____

Is diaphram in good condition? ____ Menstruation regular? ____

If there is any question patient is to return NEXT WEEK.

Jelly given: Kind ____ 1 - 2 tubes

Cash ____

Patient instructed to see physician ____ Date ____

____
Signature

An undated form titled "Patient in for Jelly" that was used by the Rochester clinic. This form as well as clinic data suggest that the clinic prescribed most patients with a diaphragm. *Scrapbook of newspaper clippings 1932-1940, Box 7, Planned Parenthood of Rochester/Syracuse Region Collection, D.325, Rare Books, Special Collections, & Preservation, River Campus Libraries, University of Rochester.*

provided they were used correctly by the patient. In *The Moral Property of Women*, Linda Gordon indicates that "the diaphragm was the most effective available contraceptive in the 1930s and certainly ought to have been offered to every birth control patient."[49] Andrea Tone also notes their effectiveness but is more hesitant to call the diaphragm reliable: "In practice, the diaphragm was 80 percent effective after a year of use, making it safer than other methods but not, by any account, infallible."[50] Tone also points out that because diaphragms were reusable, they had to be washed by hand—a task that would have been difficult for a family without access to running water.[51] For Rochester's doctors, these concerns seem to have been outweighed by the device's relative effectiveness and a hope that women would use their diaphragms correctly. In addition to these factors, diaphragms also had support from birth control proponents such as Margaret Sanger; this helped make them popular in households across the country. Tone mentions that Sanger's clinic in Brooklyn almost exclusively used the Mensinga diaphragm, a physician-fitted device made in Holland that had to be smuggled across the Canadian border.[52] There is no evidence to suggest that the Rochester clinic used similar methods to obtain their devices. Instead, "all supplies distributed to patients [at the Rochester clinic] are purchased and paid for by physicians. . . . Supplies may be dispensed only upon doctor's prescription and no advice of a medical nature is given by anyone other than the doctor."[53] To abide by state laws regarding the dispensing of contraceptives, doctors at

Devices Prescribed

Year	1936	1939	1940	1943
Number of New Patients	586	715	598	429
Number Prescribed Diaphragm and Jelly/Cream	545	674	554	399
Number Prescribed Condoms and Jelly	13	9	13	4
Number Prescribed Jelly Alone	1	1	0	1
Number Prescribed Cervi-Cap with Jelly	0	18	0	22
Miscellaneous	18	13	31	3

the clinic had to buy and distribute all devices themselves. Consequently, the availability of devices could also be a determining factor, although it is not known exactly how the Rochester physicians acquired their supplies or how much they cost.

The common prescription of the diaphragm in Rochester countered a somewhat typical line of thinking during the 1920s and 1930s that diaphragms were too complicated for underprivileged women to use effectively. Eugenicists in particular believed that lower-income individuals were uneducated and thus would not use birth control correctly.[54] Although there is no evidence to suggest that members of the Rochester clinic followed this line of thinking, reading material they would have engaged with at the time espoused these sentiments. During the 1930s, the clinic, or perhaps its physicians, subscribed to a periodical published by The Birth Control Clinical Research Bureau, a precursor to Planned Parenthood. The clinic's archival records include fourteen editions of the journal from 1936 to 1937, and a scrapbook in the collection contains a 1939 article that Ruth Backus wrote for the publication. In a 1936 article, *The Journal of Contraception* recommended that clinics send patients home with an instruction slip on how to use their new contraceptive device: "No matter how attentive the woman may be during the consultation with the physician, or how careful and explicit the instructions given her by the nurse, she is apt to

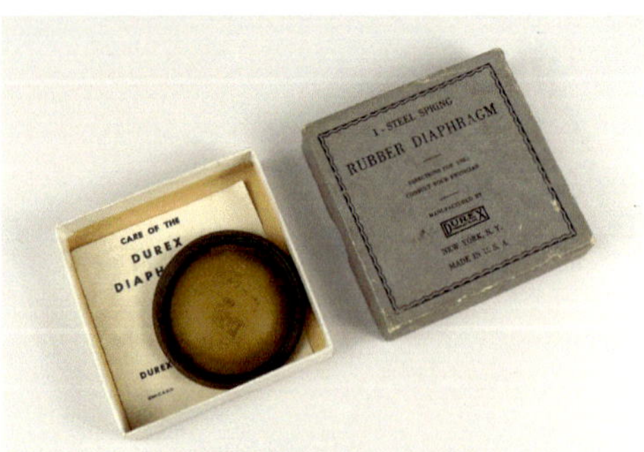

Durex brand rubber diaphragm circa 1938–1940. Diaphragms were a popular form of contraceptive in the early twentieth century but are still in use today. They provide a physical barrier to insemination, and they were often prescribed along with a spermicidal gel. *Division of Medicine and Science, National Museum of American History, Smithsonian Institution.*

forget some detail and become confused when she arrives home."[55] The article is heavy with eugenic and misogynistic sentiments, but the recommendation to give patients written instructions on how to properly use their birth control device is not inherently bad. There are no extant records suggesting whether Rochester followed the recommendation of the *Journal*, but the clinic seems to have had a low failure rate resulting from improper use of the device. The clinic saw a total of 103 unplanned pregnancies in 1939, but only six of these were because of "improper use."[56] Two years later, only fourteen of the 115 unplanned pregnancies resulted from the same reason.[57] Meanwhile, 1943 saw seventy-five unplanned pregnancies, but only nine were due to incorrect usage.[58] Clearly, doctors at the Rochester clinic had little reason to believe that their patients were too uneducated to use their devices correctly, especially considering that these numbers were well under the 20 percent failure rate noted by Tone.

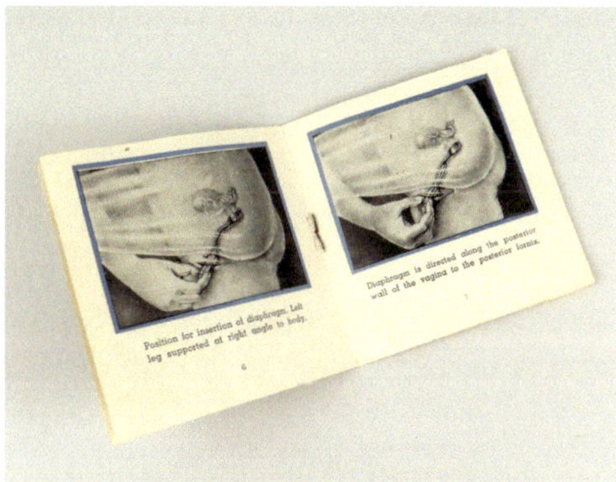

Though not always included, this set of instructions has a pair of diagrams demonstrating the proper method of inserting a diaphragm. These diagrams were part of the instructions that came with Ortho brand rubber diaphragms between 1941 and 1945. *Division of Medicine and Science, National Museum of American History, Smithsonian Institution.*

The diaphragm was not the only contraceptive method in use during this time, nor the only one the Rochester clinic prescribed. Compared to other options, diaphragms were fairly expensive, making other methods potentially more attractive to those in the working class. Tone writes that "excluding the costs of a medical consultation, the going rate for a diaphragm and a companion tube of jelly ranged from four to six dollars in the mid-1930s.[59] In contrast, a dollar purchased a dozen suppositories, ten foaming tablets, a dozen condoms, or, most alluring of all, up to three two-ounce douching units."[60] Considering that Rochester clinic patients paid at most three dollars per visit, they received a significant discount for their contraceptives. However, these cost barriers meant that for much of the general public, or those who did not go to clinics, other methods would have been more cost effective. At the Rochester clinic, the other birth control methods that women received included condoms, cervical caps, sponges and jelly or foam, or the "safe period."[61] These methods were also fairly common across the country in the 1930s and 1940s. Sometimes, clinics from a given state favored some options over others due to unique circumstances. Schoen notes in *Choices & Coercion* that spermicidal foam powder had widespread use in North Carolina during the late 1930s and early 1940s as lower-income women were used as test subjects for the new technology.[62] One might expect the Rochester clinic's preferred prescribed method to mirror that of towns and cities across New York State. However, in a 1947 survey, 27 percent of middle-class families in New York reported using diaphragms and jelly as their contraceptive, while only 2.6 percent of working-class couples did the same.[63] Their widespread use in Rochester, then, is a bit rare and demonstrates that the clinic chose to use an effective method that was potentially more costly over one that might have been cheaper, but also less successful. The women who received diaphragms from the clinic at either no or low cost certainly benefited from this decision as well as from other choices staff and volunteers made to ensure a high level of care.

Opposition to Birth Control

During the 1930s, birth control became a widely supported practice in the United States. According to a 1936 survey of 100,000 Americans, 70 percent of the population, and a majority in every state, were in favor of medical birth control.[64] However, large segments of the population opposed contraceptive access—one of the most significant groups being Catholics. Catholicism has historically had a strong and well-documented opposition to birth control practices, and during the 1930s the Church took a public stance on a national level against contraceptives.[65] On a smaller scale, local clinics faced opposition from the churches within their community, and in Rochester this antagonism was particularly powerful.

At the time the clinic was established, Rochester had a significant Catholic population. According to a 1926 national survey of church attendance, Rochester was home to 188 religious organizations boasting a total membership of 178,340 people.[66] This figure included 37 Roman Catholic churches with 92,079 parishioners, making the Roman Catholic Church by far the largest religious body in the city during the late 1920s.[67] Local census records also show a large number of Catholic immigrants in the same period. While the census of this era did not specifically track religious affiliation, inferences can be drawn based on the originating countries of polled residents. According to the 1930 census, there were 74,696 "foreign-born whites" (i.e., largely European immigrants) living in Rochester.[68] The largest share of immigrants, by far, hailed from Italy,

Rochester Population by Race, 1930

Race	Number	Percentage of Total Population
Total Population*	328,132	100%
Native white	250,598	76.4%
Foreign-born white	74,696	22.8%
Black	2,679	0.82%
Chinese	47	0.014%
Japanese	97	0.029%
Indigenous	9	0.0027%

* From U.S. Census Bureau, Fifteenth Census of the United States: 1930. 292, 297.

a predominantly Catholic country. Of the total foreign-born white population of 74,696, there were 23,935 Italian immigrants, who constituted 32 percent of the European immigrant population and 7.3 percent of the city's overall population.[69] Additionally, of the 123,163 "native white of foreign or mixed parentage" residents (i.e., second-generation immigrants), 31,478 people were born to Italian parents.[70] While Rochester also welcomed Catholic immigrants from other countries during this period, Italians undoubtedly formed the bulk of the city's foreign-born Catholic population during the 1930s and 1940s.

Although not all Catholics were against contraceptives, the Catholic population in Rochester did represent a significant oppositional bloc to the efforts of the Monroe County Birth Control League. Many early members wrote in their recollections about the antagonism the clinic faced from the Catholic Church as an organization, as well as from individual Catholic Rochesterians. In an undated letter about her time spent working with the clinic, Marjorie Harris Reynolds began by stating that "I have hesitated to set down my memories of the 1930s because the most vivid of them seem to show my dismay at the way the Catholic Church imposed the choice of abstinence or pregnancy on its people."[71] Reynolds proceeded to write five pages critiquing how the Rochester Catholic Church reacted to the clinic's existence, noting that many women were either deterred from going to the clinic because of their Church's opposition or were condemned for having gone and refused to return for a follow-up visit.[72] She concluded her account by noting that "the Public Health houses and other social workers were forbidden to give any information on Birth Control [*sic*] or the address of the clinic to even the most desperately in need mothers for fear of offending the Catholics. Not even to Protestants were they allowed to give information."[73] Reynolds's frustration and anger at the

Church is tangible in her writings; clearly it was difficult for her to see women unable to access life-changing medical information and devices because of the Church's condemnation of contraceptives. The fact that social workers avoided giving women contraceptive information because they were worried about "offending the Catholics," as Reynolds points out, suggests the considerable influence the Church held in Rochester during this time and that people of all religious backgrounds were affected by its views.

Rochester Catholics also expressed their opposition to the birth control movement at the state and federal levels. A newspaper article from January 1934—reporting on eight local women who attended the annual meeting of the New York State Birth Control Federation in New York City—noted that the meeting also drew members from the Rochester Parish Solidarity Union. Representing more than 10,000 Catholic women, the RPSU members attended the event to protest two birth control bills then being deliberated in Congress.[74] While it is surprising that this group was given a platform to speak at an annual meeting for a birth control organization, the occurrence offers additional evidence of the extent of anti-contraceptive sentiment among Rochester's Catholic population. Although volunteer recollections only mention antagonism from "the Church," rather than from Catholic women specifically, this incident makes it clear that there was a large population of Catholic individuals in Rochester who were aligned with the Church's beliefs in opposing birth control.

In some cases, the Catholic community's hostility toward birth control worked in the clinic's favor. Dr. Saul Moress wrote in his recollections that "the *Catholic Courier* gave us much criticism and adverse publicity, which re-acted in our favor. Soon, some 60% of our patients were Catholic women who had learned of our existence through the paper."[75] The exact article to which Moress is referring is unknown, but a strong contender is a series of articles published in the *Courier* on January 16, 1935. The front-page headline, "Launch Race Suicide Drive Here," was followed by various pieces discussing who "birth controllers" were, the ethics of birth control, and the Monroe County Birth Control League.[76] One article about a speaker the League was hosting opened with the line: "In a bold and open stroke designed to stir up enough public interest to raise a war chest of $5,000 to carry on their 'race suicide' activities for 1936, the Monroe County Birth Control League this week is presenting to Rochesterians Mrs. Thomas N. Hepburn, a national champion of the cause."[77] If this is indeed one of the articles to which Moress was alluding, it is impressive that so many Catholic women were able to look past such strongly worded language and view

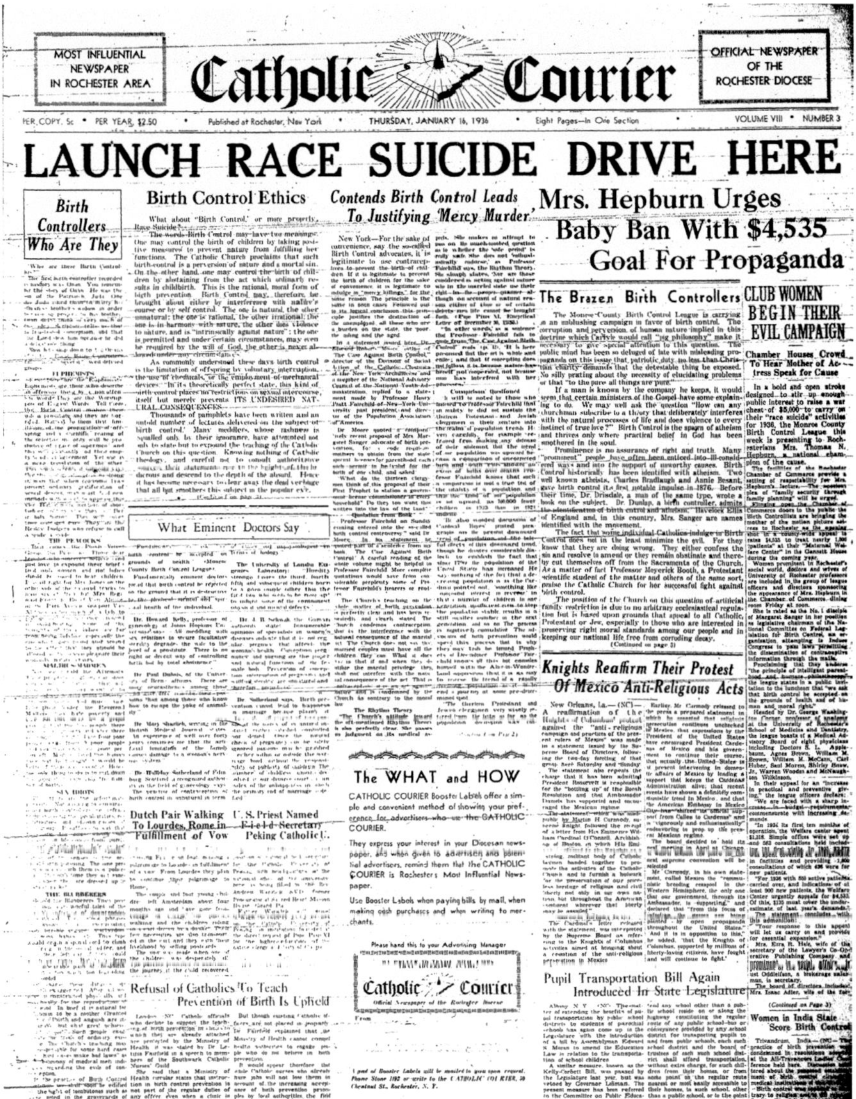

MOST INFLUENTIAL NEWSPAPER IN ROCHESTER AREA

Catholic Courier

OFFICIAL NEWSPAPER OF THE ROCHESTER DIOCESE

PER COPY, 5c • PER YEAR, $2.50 • Published at Rochester, New York • THURSDAY, JANUARY 16, 1936 • Eight Pages—In One Section • VOLUME VIII • NUMBER 3

LAUNCH RACE SUICIDE DRIVE HERE

Birth Controllers Who Are They

Birth Control Ethics

Contends Birth Control Leads To Justifying 'Mercy Murder'

Mrs. Hepburn Urges Baby Ban With $4,535 Goal For Propaganda

The Brazen Birth Controllers

CLUB WOMEN BEGIN THEIR EVIL CAMPAIGN

Chamber Houses Crowd To Hear Mother of Actress Speak for Cause

What Eminent Doctors Say

Knights Reaffirm Their Protest Of Mexico Anti-Religious Acts

Dutch Pair Walking To Lourdes, Rome in Fulfillment of Vow

U. S. Priest Named Field Secretary Peking Catholic U.

The WHAT and HOW

CATHOLIC COURIER Booster Labels offer a simple and convenient method of showing your preference for advertisers who use the CATHOLIC COURIER.

They express your interest in your Diocesan newspaper, and when given to advertisers and potential advertisers, remind them that the CATHOLIC COURIER is Rochester's Most Influential Newspaper.

Use Booster Labels when paying bills by mail, when making cash purchases and when writing to merchants.

Refusal of Catholics To Teach Prevention of Birth Is Upheld

Pupil Transportation Bill Again Introduced In State Legislature

Women in India State Score Birth Control

The Rochester-based newspaper *The Catholic Courier* was one of the most outspoken critics of the clinic. However, its coverage might have inadvertently advertised the clinic to Catholic Rochesterians. *The Catholic Courier*, 16 January 1936. *NYS Historic Newspapers. https://nyshistoricnewspapers.org/?a=d&d=cc19360116-01.1.1&srpos=3&e=-------en-20-cc-1--txt-txIN-%22birth+control+league%22---------*

the clinic as a beneficial resource.[78] Or perhaps it speaks to their desperation to manage their fertility during the difficult economic circumstances of the Great Depression, regardless of the Church's opinion. Regardless of individual motivations, however, Moress's memories align fairly well with the clinic records that are available. In 1938, 54 percent of the clinic's patients were Catholic, 43 percent were Protestant, and 3 percent were Jewish.[79] By 1939, the share of Catholic patients had shrunk slightly, to 52 percent.[80] It should be noted that this majority share of Catholic patients was probably not a direct result of the article Dr. Moress remembered, but more likely was due to the large percentage of Catholic immigrants in Rochester. As Ruth Backus noted in *The Journal of Contraception* in 1939, "nearly one third of the patients [accepted between the clinic's opening and January 1, 1939] were Italian by birth or parentage."[81] It is likely that the clinic served other immigrant populations as well, especially given the financial challenges many recent arrivals faced and endured, but the records do not contain specific demographic information beyond race.[82] Regardless of immigration status, it is notable that despite strong opposition from the local Catholic Church, such a large percentage of Catholic women still sought assistance from the clinic.

Catholic opposition to contraceptives affected clinics across the country as well as actions taken by those involved with the organized birth control movement. Maria Anderson's study of Houston's first clinic notes that the Bishop of Galveston wrote articles in the *Houston Post* during WWII "disparag[ing] America's loss of religion and Planned Parenthood's role in bringing it about."[83] As in Rochester, Catholic authorities in Texas were vocal about their opposition to such clinics.[84] Writing about the broader American response to birth control promotion in the 1920s and 1930s, Linda Gordon notes that "the most powerful organized opposition to birth control came from the Catholic Church. . . . Catholic women at this time consistently used birth control less and attended clinics less than Jewish or Protestant women; nevertheless, many working-class Catholic women used contraceptives."[85] Although some Catholic women across the country used birth control during this period, their usage rates were lower than that of Jewish or Protestant women, which counters the trend in Rochester, where the majority of clinic patients were Catholic. This may have been due to the religious affiliation of the clinic's targeted clientele or the city's strong Catholic bent, but it is also possible that the volunteers who ran the Monroe County Birth Control League may have known how to reach area Catholics better than clinic employees in other locations. Gordon also observes that at one New York City clinic with a predominantly working-class Italian Catholic clientele, 64.5 percent of patients had used birth control prior to their consultation. At a different clinic with a predominantly Protestant patient base, about 90 percent had used birth control before.[86] These statistics are lower than those reported by the Rochester clinic for prior contraceptive use. In Ruth Backus's speech "The Extra-Mural Center," she stated that "among the 2,700 women already advised at the Maternal Consultation Center in Rochester, 97 percent had previously used some method of birth control," although these were often methods not supported by those in the medical profession.[87] Backus did not offer any breakdown of this statistic by religious affiliation, but this figure combined with the majority Catholic clientele of the Rochester clinic implies that Rochester women were unique in their birth control usage, both before and after visiting the clinic. This bucking of a larger trend can perhaps be explained simply: women who wanted birth control were likely to take advantage of the resources they had to get it, regardless of outside opinion. An anecdote from Margaret Sanger about the first day of operations for her Brooklyn clinic, discussed in Gordon's book, demonstrates this point as well: "As many Catholics came as Jews. When Sanger asked one Catholic woman what she would say to the priest at confession, the woman replied, 'It's none of his business. My husband has a weak heart and works only four days a week. He gets twelve dollars, and we can barely live on it now. We have enough children.'"[88] Certainly, many Rochester women must have felt similarly, given that almost every patient who came to the clinic had previously used birth control, and a little more than half of these women were Catholic themselves.

Significantly, Italian immigrants across the country demonstrated shifting attitudes regarding family planning in the early decades of the twentieth century. Although immigrants in this era, especially Catholic ones, often had higher birthrates than native-born white populations, these rates were comparatively lower than those in their country of origin.[89] Research by John Briggs illustrates that this trend was already taking shape in Rochester at the turn of the twentieth century: Italian-born residents demonstrated lower fertility rates than women who remained in their home villages.[90] In the 1920s and 1930s, the United States witnessed a considerable decline in the birth rate, owing in no small part to the fact that foreign-born women were having fewer children than their immigrant predecessors. Second-generation Americans further contributed to this decline.[91] Italian immigrant women tended to marry later than their peers back home, which necessarily influenced their fertility rate, but they were also controlling their family sizes to a greater extent than their peers in Italy.[92] Italian-born women were consistently having fewer children than if they had stayed in Italy, suggesting that while Catholic attitudes were certainly influential, other factors also affected how women chose to engage with contraception.

Catholic opposition to the birth control movement was a trend that extended beyond any one city or region. This issue directly affected Rochester in determining how the clinic operated, the population it was able to serve, and the personal beliefs of those who were involved with the Monroe County Birth Control League. Despite the national prevalence of such opposition, however, Rochester's experience suggests that it was perhaps not as pervasive or as persuasive as it otherwise might appear to have been.

Conclusion

The birth control movement of the early twentieth century shaped the lives of many people across the United States. As contraception became easier to access, more families began to take advantage of it to prevent unwanted pregnancies, especially during the economically challenging times of the Great Depression. For members of the working class, however, birth control access was partly dependent on clinics that would provide contraception at low or no cost. The early clinics these women frequented were often locally founded and managed, with clinic operators directly engaging with the communities they were serving. Rochester's first clinic, established in 1934, had an immediate impact. It quickly expanded, relocating to a larger facility in 1937. By 1943, it was holding more than 200 "sessions," or counseling days, per year.[93] The segment of Rochester's population it served was not immense, but its effects were certainly felt by those who used the clinic for their family planning needs.

Though it was locally run, the Rochester clinic did not exist in a vacuum. Between 1937 and 1940, the number of birth control clinics in the United States jumped from 357 to 800.[94] These clinics witnessed national trends regarding both the services and the devices they offered, and they collectively experienced resistance to the nationwide birth control movement. Rochester, in many ways, both adhered to these trends and broke away from them. The clinic's predominantly working-class, married clientele mirrored the patient demographics of birth control clinics across the country. The diaphragm—by far the most popular method prescribed by the Rochester clinic—was also in use across the United States in this era, despite concerns from some that it was an unfit device for underprivileged individuals. Yet the diaphragm was not commonly employed by low-income women due to cost, demonstrating that Rochester physicians chose to provide a more reliable method over one that would have been less costly and less effective. Consequently, in this respect Rochester was both part of the national trend and an outlier. The Catholic Church, which strongly opposed birth control in many areas of the country, also opposed the services of the Rochester clinic and made efforts to prevent women from accessing its resources. However, the clinic was still able to serve a sizeable Catholic population, counter to nationwide trends. These discrepancies beg the question of whether other early birth control clinics might also reveal unique patterns if examined on a smaller scale.

When people are looking to get involved in a cause, they are often advised to start on a local level—where they can make the greatest difference. In Rochester, and likely in many other areas, the local founders, volunteers, and members of the birth control clinic were able to work on the ground to help those with whom they shared a city. They did not come from the same socioeconomic classes as the clinic's patients, but they would have understood Rochester's dynamics and how to best reach those affected by local phenomena. Examining these early facilities from a local perspective—before they became affiliated with larger groups—elucidates trends that might otherwise be invisible and suggests that the history of early birth control clinics in the United States is far more multifaceted than previously assumed. ■

1 Following the language used during this era, as well as that of other scholars, "birth control" will be used throughout this article exclusively to discuss contraceptive methods as opposed to other services such as sterilization and abortion. The Rochester clinic only provided contraceptive services, so abortion and sterilization, while significant parts of the larger conversation, do not factor into the clinic's work. Johanna Schoen uses similar terminology in *Choice & Coercion: Birth Control, Sterilization, and Abortion in Public Health*, dividing her book into sections on birth control (contraception), sterilization, and abortion. During its early years, the Rochester clinic's members tried to avoid using language such as "birth control" due to public resistance to these terms, preferring instead to use promotional phrases such as "every child a wanted child." However, medical literature from the time included statements such as, "the term 'birth control' denotes the prevention of conception only, and not sterilization or abortion." Therefore, the term birth control should be understood only as a reference to contraceptive methods and devices that might have been prescribed to women during this time and will be used in spite of the Rochester clinic's opposition to the phrase. From Johanna Schoen, *Choice & Coercion: Birth Control, Sterilization, and Abortion in Public Health and Welfare* (Chapel Hill: University of North Carolina Press, 2005). Reminiscences of Marcia Ellingson, 10 June

1973, Planned Parenthood of Rochester/Syracuse Region, 1973, Box 6, Folder 4, Planned Parenthood of Rochester/Syracuse Region Collection, Rare Books, Special Collections and Preservation, University of Rochester, Rochester, New York; hereafter cited as Reminiscences of Marcia Ellingson, PP of Rochester/Syracuse. "A Medical View of Birth Control," *The Journal of Contraception* 1, no. 4 (1936): 47. Accessed via Rare Books, Special Collections and Preservation, University of Rochester, Rochester, New York.

2 Clinic Records, Planned Parenthood of Rochester/Syracuse Region, 1934–1956, Box 5, Folder 1, Planned Parenthood of Rochester/Syracuse Region Collection, Rare Books, Special Collections and Preservation, University of Rochester, Rochester, New York; hereafter cited as Clinic Records, PP of Rochester/Syracuse.

3 The archival records for the clinic, which are held by the University of Rochester's Rare Books, Special Collections and Preservation library, consist primarily of compiled data sheets for different years of the clinic's operation, reminiscences from staff and volunteers, and newspaper clippings about the clinic and its functions. There are no records that discuss personal information about patients beyond compiled statistics or that include firsthand patient testimonies about their experiences at the clinic. In this article, I use the available records to better understand the motivations of the clinic founders and volunteers, while providing general information about its patients based on what limited records of them exist.

4 One of the significant aspects of Rochester's demographics during this period was that the population was almost entirely white. According to the 1930 census, Rochester had a total population of 328,132 people—including 2,679 African Americans, 47 Native Americans, 97 Chinese, and 9 Japanese citizens. Because of this, the racial demographics of the city during this time, and the ones pertinent to this study, are more closely focused on immigrant versus "native-born" white populations. See Table 1 for the population breakdowns. From US Census Bureau, *Fifteenth Census of the United States: 1930*, 277, 297.

5 Rochester's birth control clinic underwent several name changes throughout its years of operation. The clinic opened in 1934 under the operation of the Monroe County Birth Control League but referred to itself in documents by several names, including the Maternal Welfare Center and Maternal Consultation Center. Ruth H. Backus, the director of the clinic from 1934 to 1954, discussed in her 1964 publication, *From the Cradle*, the difficulty they had in deciding on a name: "Due to the fact that we had no license to operate a 'clinic' nor any hope of obtaining one, we had to avoid that word. Almost everyone wanted to avoid the controversial words, 'Birth control.' . . . We started off with the innocuous name of Welfare Center, later changed to Maternal Welfare Center." Backus noted that the clinic changed its name to the Maternal Consultation Center following its first move. The clinic was still operating under the title Maternal Consultation Center in 1945, but operations had by then switched to the Monroe County League for Planned Parenthood. Later in the 1940s, the clinic was rebranded as the Planned Parenthood League of Rochester and Monroe County. For the sake of clarity in this article, the clinic will be referred to by its first title of the Monroe County Birth Control League or just "the clinic." This language would not have been favored by the community organizers who operated the clinic during this time, but it is the best descriptor of the services it provided. From Clinic Records, 1932, 1936, PP of Rochester/Syracuse.; Ruth H. Backus, *From the Cradle*, 1964, Box 6, Folder 2, Planned Parenthood of Rochester/Syracuse Region Collection, Rare Books, Special Collections and Preservation, University of Rochester, Rochester, New York; hereafter cited as Backus, *From the Cradle,* PP of Rochester/Syracuse.; Volunteer Manual, PP of Rochester/Syracuse.

6 "Birth Control Unit Picks New Officers," *Democrat and Chronicle*, October 30, 1935; "Reynolds, Marjorie Harris (Oddleifson)," *Democrat and Chronicle*, June 22, 1989.

7 Reminiscences of Marcia Ellingson, PP of Rochester/Syracuse.

8 Rickie Solinger, *Pregnancy and Power: A Short History of Reproductive Politics in America* (New York: New York University Press, 2005), 105.

9 Linda Gordon, *The Moral Property of Women: A History of Birth Control Politics in America* (Champaign: University of Illinois Press, 2002), ProQuest Ebook Central, 203.
10 Solinger, *Pregnancy and Power*, 104.
11 Gordon, *The Moral Property of Women*, 201.
12 Andrea Tone, *Devices and Desires: A History of Contraceptives in America* (New York: Hill and Wang, 2001), 82.
13 Schoen, *Choice & Coercion*, 35.
14 Maria Helen Anderson, "Private choices vs. public voices: The history of Planned Parenthood in Houston" (1998). Diss., Rice University, https://hdl.handle.net/1911/19239, 7. While the Cleveland case study is not used in this article, it is an excellent reference for those who are interested in reading more about the history of local birth control activism. See Jimmy Elaine Wilkinson Meyer, *Any Friend of the Movement: Networking for Birth Control, 1920–1940*, (Columbus: Ohio State University Press, 2004).
15 Anderson, "Private choices vs. public voices," 3–4.
16 Anderson, "Private choices vs. public voices," 7.
17 Backus, *From the Cradle*, PP of Rochester/Syracuse.
18 Backus, *From the Cradle*, PP of Rochester/Syracuse.
19 Much of the language used by the volunteers raises ideas of maternalism, or a desire by the wealthy to aid those whom they viewed as lesser than them. Nothing in the archival record supports the idea that these women felt this way toward the clientele of the clinic, but it's impossible to know their true motivations based on the sources available. Backus, *From the Cradle*, PP of Rochester/Syracuse.
20 This rent is roughly $593.84 in 2024 dollars. Calculated on May 15, 2024, from https://www.usinflationcalculator.com/. From Backus, *From the Cradle*, PP of Rochester/Syracuse.
21 Reminiscences of Ruth Briggs, 7 June 1973, Planned Parenthood of Rochester/Syracuse Region, 1973, Box 6, Folder 2, Planned Parenthood of Rochester/Syracuse Region Collection, Rare Books, Special Collections and Preservation, University of Rochester, Rochester, New York; hereafter cited as Reminiscences of Ruth Briggs, PP of Rochester/Syracuse.
22 Clinic Records, 1934, PP of Rochester/Syracuse Region.
23 "Birth Control Needed, Says Woman Doctor," *Democrat and Chronicle*, November 1, 1934.
24 Reminiscences of Miggie Baum, June 1973, Planned Parenthood of Rochester/Syracuse Region, 1973, Box 6, Folder 4, Planned Parenthood of Rochester/Syracuse Region Collection, Rare Books, Special Collections and Preservation, University of Rochester, Rochester, New York; hereafter cited as Reminiscences of Miggie Baum, PP of Rochester/Syracuse.
25 An undated handwritten note from Ruth H. Backus at the bottom of this document states that this constitution was "supposed to be our policy but wasn't!" However, the clinic records demonstrate an adherence to many of its principles. Backus notes in *From the Cradle* that Dr. William Brown wrote this document.
26 Clinic Constitution from First Scrap Book, 1932–1940, Planned Parenthood of Rochester/Syracuse Region, 1934, Box 7, Planned Parenthood of Rochester/Syracuse Region Collection, Rare Books, Special Collections and Preservation, University of Rochester, Rochester, New York; hereafter cited as Clinic Constitution, PP of Rochester/Syracuse.
27 Anderson, "Private choices vs. public voices," 7.
28 For many years, including 1940, women were refused treatment because they were "pregnant on coming." Clinic Records, 1940, PP of Rochester/Syracuse.
29 Reminiscences of Ruth H. Backus, 26 June 1982, Planned Parenthood of Rochester/Syracuse Region, 1982, Box 6, Folder 5, Planned Parenthood of Rochester/Syracuse Region Collection, Rare Books, Special Collections and Preservation, University of Rochester, Rochester, New York; hereafter cited as Reminiscences of Ruth H. Backus, PP of Rochester/Syracuse.
30 Gordon, *The Moral Property of Women*, 226.

31 Clinic Records, 1939, 1940, 1943, PP of Rochester/Syracuse. See Table 2 for detailed information about the financial eligibility breakdown.

32 Archival documents are not specific about what constituted a "valid health reason" to seek contraception. However, Backus states that the first four patients had "economic problems but serious health ones as well. Otherwise they could not have been accepted, as health reasons for giving contraceptive advice had to be written on the chart." She also states that child spacing eventually counted as a valid health reason, but this took "some time." From Backus, *From the Cradle*, PP of Rochester/Syracuse. Clinic Records, 1939, 1940, 1943, PP of Rochester/Syracuse.

33 Clinic Constitution, 1934, PP of Rochester/Syracuse.

34 Clinic Records, 1939, 1940, 1943, PP of Rochester/Syracuse. See Table 3, for detailed information about the financial breakdown. Between $0.22 and $22.33 in 2024 dollars. Calculated from https://www.usinflationcalculator.com/ on March 13, 2024.

35 $433.57 in 2024 dollars. Calculated from https://www.usinflationcalculator.com/ on March 13, 2024; Clinic Records, 1940, PP of Rochester/Syracuse.

36 The records use this language without clarifying what these terms mean. It is unknown if "self/partially-supporting" meant that patients paid for household expenses in either whole or part, or if they supported themselves without governmental assistance. It is also unclear if this is referring to their status as a single- or dual-income household, but given the clinic's refusal to help single women, this language likely is applicable only to married women. From Clinic Records, 1943, PP of Rochester/Syracuse.

37 Clinic Records, 1939, 1940, 1943, PP of Rochester/Syracuse.

38 Reminiscences of Florence H. King, 26 June 1973, Planned Parenthood of Rochester/Syracuse Region, 1973, Box 6, Folder 4, Planned Parenthood of Rochester/Syracuse Region Collection, Rare Books, Special Collections and Preservation, University of Rochester, Rochester, New York. Hereafter cited as Reminiscences of Florence H. King, PP of Rochester/Syracuse.

39 Reminiscences of Marcia Ellingson, PP of Rochester/Syracuse.

40 "The Extra-Mural Center," speech by Ruth H. Backus, June 19, 1939, Planned Parenthood of Rochester/Syracuse Region, 1973, Box 7, Planned Parenthood of Rochester/Syracuse Region Collection, Rare Books, Special Collections and Preservation, University of Rochester, Rochester, New York; hereafter cited as "The Extra-Mural Center," PP of Rochester/Syracuse.

41 For more on the concepts of the "undeserving poor" and "deserving poor," see Michael B. Katz, *The Undeserving Poor: From the War on Poverty to the War on Welfare* (New York: Pantheon Books, 1989).

42 Anderson, "Private choices vs. public voices," 16–17.

43 Gordon, *The Moral Property of Women*, 148.

44 Tone, *Devices and Desires*, 74.

45 Reminiscences of Dr. Saul Moress, undated, Planned Parenthood of Rochester/Syracuse Region, undated, Box 6, Folder 4, Planned Parenthood of Rochester/Syracuse Region Collection, Rare Books, Special Collections and Preservation, University of Rochester, Rochester, New York; hereafter cited as Reminiscences of Dr. Saul Moress, PP of Rochester/Syracuse.

46 Ruth Backus, "Clinic Reports: The Maternal Consultation Center, Rochester, New York," *The Journal of Contraception* First Scrap Book, 1932–1940, Planned Parenthood of Rochester/Syracuse Region, 1939, Box 7, Planned Parenthood of Rochester/Syracuse Region Collection, Rare Books, Special Collections and Preservation, University of Rochester, Rochester, New York.

47 "Patient in for Jelly" form, First Scrap Book, 1932–1940, Planned Parenthood of Rochester/Syracuse Region, undated, Box 7, Planned Parenthood of Rochester/Syracuse Region Collection, Rare Books, Special Collections and Preservation, University of Rochester, Rochester, New York; hereafter cited as "Patient in for Jelly," PP of Rochester/Syracuse.

48 Clinic Records, 1939, 1940, 1943, PP of Rochester/Syracuse. See Table 4 for detailed information about the devices prescribed.

49 Gordon, *The Moral Property of Women*, 217.
50 Tone, *Devices and Desires*, 154.
51 Tone, *Devices and Desires*, 154.
52 Tone, *Devices and Desires*, 121, 126.
53 Volunteer Manual, 1945, PP of Rochester/Syracuse.
54 Eugenics is a term with broad application, but it generally describes people who believed that certain groups were superior to others, whether that was based on racial, class, or other characteristics. A key part of many eugenicist beliefs was to encourage people from certain groups to have children and/or to prevent those in other groups from the same. Because of this, eugenics are a significant part of the national conversation surrounding birth control during the period under discussion, although there is no evidence that the Rochester volunteers subscribed to eugenic beliefs themselves. Gordon, *The Moral Property of Women*, 216.
55 "Instruction Slips," *The Journal of Contraception* 1, no. 4 (1936): 56. Accessed via Rare Books, Special Collections and Preservation, University of Rochester, Rochester, New York.
56 Clinic Records, 1939, PP of Rochester/Syracuse.
57 Clinic Records, 1941, PP of Rochester/Syracuse.
58 Clinic Records, 1943, PP of Rochester/Syracuse.
59 Four to six dollars would be between $90.61 and $135.91 in 2024 dollars, with 1935 being used as the sample year. Calculated from https://www.usinflationcalculator.com/ on March 14, 2024.
60 Tone, *Devices and Desires*, 155. Compared to the $4.00 to $6.00 rate for a diaphragm and jelly in the above footnote, $1.00 in 1935 would be equivalent to $22.65 in 2024 dollars. Calculated from https://www.usinflationcalculator.com/ on March 14, 2024.
61 The "safe period" is a birth control method where a couple only has sex when a woman is unlikely to be ovulating. This method requires no prescription or device but does require women to track their menstrual cycles to determine when they are ovulating. This method was only "prescribed" to one woman in 1936. From Clinic Records, 1936, PP of Rochester/Syracuse.
62 Schoen, *Choice & Coercion*, 33.
63 Tone, *Devices and Desires*, 153.
64 Tone, *Devices and Desires*, 152.
65 Gordon, *The Moral Property of Women*, 228.
66 United States Department of Commerce, *Religious Bodies: 1926*, Volume I (Washington DC: United States Government Printing Office, 1930), 525.
67 United States Department of Commerce, *Religious Bodies: 1926*, Volume I, 526.
68 US Census Bureau, *Fifteenth Census of the United States: 1930*, 300.
69 Rochester's total population in 1930 was 328,132. From US Census Bureau, *Fifteenth Census of the United States: 1930*, 277, 300–301.
70 "Native white" was a term used by the Census Bureau during this time to indicate people who were of European descent but born in the United States. This should not be confused with Indigenous populations. US Census Bureau, *Fifteenth Census of the United States: 1930*, 304.
71 Reminiscences of Marjorie Harris Reynolds, undated, Planned Parenthood of Rochester/Syracuse Region, undated, Box 6, Folder 4, Planned Parenthood of Rochester/Syracuse Region Collection, Rare Books, Special Collections and Preservation, University of Rochester, Rochester, New York; hereafter cited as Reminiscences of Marjorie Harris Reynolds, PP of Rochester/Syracuse.
72 Reminiscences of Marjorie Harris Reynolds, PP of Rochester/Syracuse.
73 Reminiscences of Marjorie Harris Reynolds, PP of Rochester/Syracuse.
74 "8 Attend Meeting on Birth Control," First Scrap Book, January 1934, Planned Parenthood of Rochester/Syracuse Region, 1934, Box 7, Planned Parenthood of Rochester/Syracuse Region Collection, Rare Books, Special Collections and Preservation, University of Rochester, Rochester, New York; hereafter cited as "8 Attend Meeting on Birth Control," PP of Rochester/Syracuse.

75 Reminiscences of Dr. Saul Moress, PP of Rochester/Syracuse.

76 The phrase "race suicide" was employed by eugenicists to suggest what would happen if the members of "desirable" groups voluntarily chose to not have children. In this case, the headline is suggesting that if Catholics chose to use contraceptives it would lead to the end of the Catholic population. From "Launch Race Suicide Drive Here," *The Catholic Courier*, January 16, 1935, https://nyshistoricnewspapers.org/?a=d&d=cc19360116-01.1.1&srpos=3&e=-------en-20-cc-1--txt-txIN-%22birth+control+league%22--------- (accessed November 7, 2023).

77 "Club Women Begin Their Evil Campaign," *The Catholic Courier*, January 16, 1935, https://nyshistoricnewspapers.org/?a=d&d=cc19360116-01.1.1&srpos=3&e=-------en-20-cc-1--txt-txIN-%22birth+control+league%22--------- (accessed November 7, 2023).

78 Italian and Polish Catholic immigrants likely didn't read the *Catholic Courier*, but rather publications in their own languages. The paper proved popular with English-speaking Catholics, however.

79 Clinic Records, 1938, PP of Rochester/Syracuse.

80 Clinic Records, 1939, 1943, PP of Rochester/Syracuse.

81 "Clinic Reports: The Maternal Consultation Center, Rochester, New York." *The Journal of Contraception*, October 1939, accessed via Rare Books, Special Collections and Preservation, University of Rochester, Rochester, New York.

82 The clinic recorded race in three categories: "White," "Negro," and either "Red" or "Other." During the three years racial information was recorded (1939, 1940, and 1943), only 22 of the 1,742 patients fell into a category other than "White." Although race is often an important part of the discussion surrounding birth control accessibility in the United States, in Rochester both the BIPOC population and those aided by the clinic were too small to result in any real conclusions. From Clinic Records, 1939, 1940, 1943, PP of Rochester/Syracuse.

83 Anderson, "Private choices vs. public voices," 102.

84 The feelings of individual Catholics or how this might have affected clinic clientele in Houston aren't addressed in Anderson's work.

85 Gordon, *The Moral Property of Women*, 228.

86 Gordon, *The Moral Property of Women*, 228.

87 "The Extra-Mural Center," PP of Rochester/Syracuse.

88 Gordon, *The Moral Property of Women*, 157.

89 Diane C. Vecchio, *Merchants, Midwives, and Laboring Women: Italian Migrants in Urban America* (Urbana: University of Illinois Press, 2006), 94.

90 John Briggs, "Fertility and Cultural Change among Families in Italy and America," *American Historical Review* 91, no. 5 (December 1986): 1129–45.

91 Nancy F. Cott, *The Grounding of Modern Feminism* (New Haven, CT: Yale University Press, 1987), 167; J. Davis Hacker and Evan Roberts, "Fertility Decline in the United States, 1850–1930: New Evidence from Complete-Count Datasets," *Ann Demogr Hist* (Paris) 138, no. 2 (June 2019): 143–77.

92 Vecchio, *Merchants, Midwives, and Laboring Women*, 94.

93 Clinic Records, 1943, PP of Rochester/Syracuse.

94 Tone, *Devices and Desires*, 153.

REVIEW ESSAY

Your Children Are Very Greatly in Danger: School Segregation in Rochester, New York

by Justin Murphy. Ithaca, NY: Cornell University Press, 2022.

Just Action: How to Challenge Segregation Enacted Under the Color of Law

by Richard Rothstein and Leah Rothstein.
New York: Liveright Publishing Corporation, 2023.

Richard D. Deverell

Justin Murphy's *Your Children Are Very Greatly in Danger: School Segregation in Rochester, New York* and Richard and Leah Rothstein's *Just Action: How to Challenge Segregation Enacted Under the Color of Law* both examine the current state of segregation in cities while offering specific advice for undoing the legacy of decades of policies designed in support of white property wealth at the expense of African Americans and other people of color. Reporter Justin Murphy has written about education and the Rochester City School District for the *Democrat and Chronicle* (Rochester, New York) since 2012.[1] His book, developed from several of the columns he wrote over the years, focuses on the school district. Father-daughter writing team Richard and Leah Rothstein both focus on race, education, and segregation in their professional activities and publications. Richard Rothstein is a Distinguished Fellow of the Economic Policy Institute and works for the NAACP Legal Defense Fund. Leah Rothstein studied Public Policy and American Studies and now consults for nonprofits, cities, and other organizations dedicated to greater housing equity.[2] The authors of both works summarize the role of residential segregation while offering radical plans to confront the structural inequalities that maintain segregation in housing and, by extension, in education.

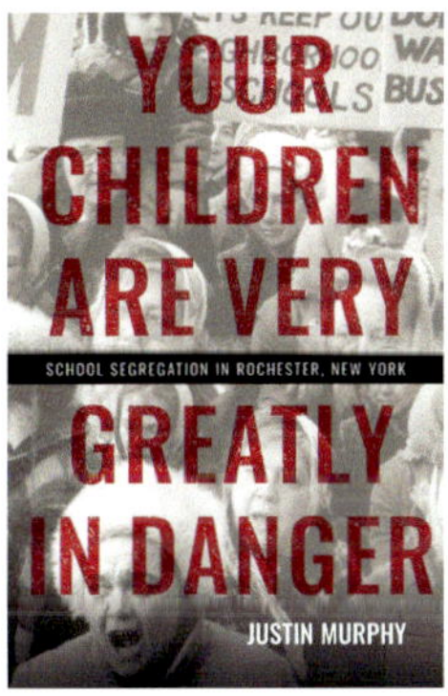

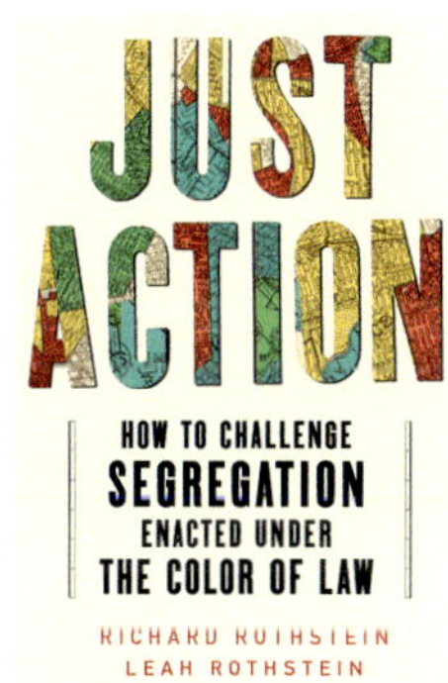

Both Murphy and the Rothsteins discuss how the conditions of segregation in education and housing are the result of government programs and the actions of individuals in several interconnected industries over the course of decades. Murphy successfully argues that the current state of Rochester, New York, city schools and the "educational disparities across the metropolitan area are attributable to explicit racial segregation and discrimination" beginning in the nineteenth century.[3] Rochester shares with most places in the United States its failure to "confront the racial and socioeconomic segregation that underlies and perpetuates its most pressing problems."[4] He specifically focuses on the role of segregation in education as underpinning these social problems, though his work connects education with segregation in housing and other aspects of life in Rochester. Although Murphy credits Rochester as the "first large school district in New York to fully desegregate," this early success belied later struggles as housing segregation worked to create a form of de facto segregation in Rochester schools, particularly in the difference between Rochester and other Monroe County school districts.[5] In their work, the Rothsteins build upon Richard Rothstein's earlier book, *The Color of Law: A Forgotten History of How Our Government Segregated America* (Liveright, 2017), to argue that segregation follows government policies designed to subsidize the growth of the white working class while excluding Black working-class families from achieving the same intergenerational wealth.[6] They note that even if the government dedicated itself to zealously enforcing antidiscrimination ordinances, such efforts could "do little to transform racial living patterns that were established fifty or one hundred years ago."[7] In support of their arguments, the authors of each book examine the long history of segregation in housing and education.

While casual readers may only consider segregation as it relates to de jure policies in the post–Civil War American South during the late nineteenth and twentieth centuries, the historiography of de facto segregation and other policies to deny people of color equal treatment in the Northern states and the American West provides a useful background for Murphy's and the Rothsteins' books. Thomas Sugrue's work focuses on the civil rights struggle in the North, arguing that protests there paralleled and eclipsed those in the South. He specifically notes of Rochester, New York, that "a broad spectrum of civil rights activists and nationalists, including Malcolm X, joined forces in protesting the city's police, who had arrested twelve members of the Nation of Islam in January" 1963.[8] Regarding housing, Sugrue argues, "The existence of all-white and all-black neighborhoods was not a fixed, timeless feature of northern life. Rather, rigid housing segregation by race was a relatively new creation."[9] While certain Northern towns enacted sundown laws (where people of color were prohibited from frequenting a given town after sunset), more common were neighborhood associations or Realtors® who limited prospective homebuyers.[10] In the West, specifically Orange County, California, the "high rate of home ownership contributed to a germinating conservative political culture."[11] This led to a political climate that highlighted individual success linked to "traditional" values.[12] Matthew Lassiter's work critically linked class with race in examining the rise of conservatism in the Sunbelt South, particularly amid 1960s' conservatives' ideological constructs of neighborhood identities.[13] He notes how Atlanta's open-schools movement pitted upwardly mobile urbanites against "reactionary rural demagogues" who were committed to maintaining the social and racial status quo.[14] Facing community efforts to rectify segregation through busing, those citizen-demagogues opposed to these actions found creative strategies in challenging the programs based on the supposed spirit of the

Brown v. Board of Education decision and the "race-neutral requirement of the U.S. Constitution."[15] Nationally, the so-called Silent Majority "obscured the divisions between working-class and middle-class white voters and defined Middle America through a suburban identity politics based on consumer status, taxpayer rights, and meritocratic individualism."[16] Finally, the process of deindustrialization, economic turbulence, and conservative attacks on welfare programs from the 1970s onward disguised "as *racial* problems the general social problems" that followed these processes, leading many whites to reinvest in elements of white identity that obscured their privilege—while criticizing people of color for suffering under these changes.[17] Segregationists thus adopted multiple policies unique to the social, political, and economic situations of each town, city, and state, with successive generations failing to realize that the makeup of their communities reflected constructed ideologies rather than natural patterns of settlement.

In *Your Children Are Very Greatly in Danger*, Murphy largely progresses chronologically in his examination of school policies in Rochester and Monroe County, touching on economic and other policies as appropriate for their influence on school attendance. He notes how Rochester enshrined segregated education in 1841, though quickly discovered the monetary cost of building and maintaining two distinct school systems based on race.[18] Through activists' efforts, Rochester quietly and grudgingly desegregated its schools in 1855, giving students "free choice of schools in 1872."[19] The northward migrations of African Americans and Latin Americans seeking work in industry and agriculture in the twentieth century began demographically changing the city, but mechanisms—including "defiant neighbors and deceitful landlords" as well as federal government policies—enforced housing segregation, leading to segregated education; many children walked to school and could not travel far beyond their immediate neighborhoods.[20] Further, Black students in Rochester's schools often lacked any Black teachers to look up to until the mid-twentieth century.[21] Even after the *Brown v. Board of Education* decision of 1954, Rochester newspapers urged "patience in its implementation."[22] Later efforts to combat segregation relied on voluntary participation and, "because the Black children were a distinct minority, the burden of assimilation, both social and academic, fell on their shoulders."[23] White flight to the suburbs ensured that the city schools remained segregated within the county.[24] This historical evidence demonstrates that segregation in the Rochester City School District has a long history, such that the voluntary half-measures in the wake of *Brown* could not rectify it. Murphy's analysis neatly complements the larger historiography of segregation, though his argument and evidence do not require prior familiarity with specific foundational texts in order to appreciate his conclusions, particularly given the narrow focus of his book.

Richard and Leah Rothstein present their evidence such that it draws upon existing scholarship and contains extensive notes for further reading. Unlike with Murphy, those readers who intend to act on the Rothsteins' suggested solutions will require further reading, but the authors intend for their book to continue the discussion that Richard Rothstein began in his previous book. The Rothsteins alternate between detailed examinations of prior legislation and policies supporting home buyers and analyses of efforts to challenge segregation. They generally structure their analyses around examinations of specific policies, progressing more or less chronologically. The Rothsteins note how various judicial rulings and policies failed to achieve the goals of desegregation. For example, they argue that the government rarely enforces the Fair Housing Act of 1968 and that such enforcement cannot undo decades of prior segregation.[25] Even efforts to increase Black homeownership face challenges as "more than a century of discriminatory zoning policies in black neighborhoods have permitted nonresidential uses, such as industry and even toxic dumps, to be placed in many black areas," thereby lowering property values so that homeowners cannot afford to sell and move to healthier neighborhoods with greater amenities.[26] Both assessments and appraisals of Black-owned properties or in majority African American communities work to homeowners' disadvantage, with those homeowners having less success in appealing the results than white homeowners with similar properties.[27] The overwhelming failure of governments to enforce anti-segregation policies, coupled with seemingly race-blind practices (for example, banks' use of credit scores in offering financing, property assessments, and appraisals) and economic investment that only furthers gentrification, combine to maintain current housing and neighborhood segregation.

Having described the magnitude of the problem, the authors of both books offer solutions to combat segregation. The Rothsteins note that the Supreme Court may afford an opportunity to enact great changes, but that these changes should not rely upon a court that may issue a different ruling when new judges ascend to the bench. To this end, they advocate for localities pushing forward policies and programs even if they may face potential judicial review, noting that failure to act simply due to fears of possible challenges does a disservice to those most in need of new policies.[28] They further list the important policies that activists must mobilize to ensure the preservation of neighborhoods' characters in the face of gentrification, including "inclusionary (mixed-income) zoning, rent control, prohibition of evictions except for just cause, prevention of security-deposit theft, limits on condominium conversions, support for community land trusts, regulation of phony home sales, and property-tax freezes."[29] They propose new programs and an expansion of government powers to prevent the loss of affordable housing, such as municipal governments purchasing rental units when owners cannot guarantee new purchasers will maintain rent control.[30] The Rothsteins also discuss educational initiatives at the local level, including one that fourth-grade teacher Shane Wiegand created in Rochester to answer students' questions about neighborhood discrimination.[31] For his part, Murphy describes how Monroe County could hypothetically expand a system like the Board of Cooperative Educational Services (BOCES) to encompass the entire county, helping to more evenly distribute the work toward desegregation while better allocating resources for special education and technical training.[32] He notes that the idea is not novel to his book, but it never gained significant support, especially once suburban districts decided to support their local tax base and later financially gain through support of limited urban-suburban programs.[33] Murphy concludes with a call for a thorough report on metropolitan reforms in education, including the possibility of creating a county school system,[34] written policies to create greater equity for suburban districts to participate in urban-suburban programs, and intensive anti-racism training in all Rochester-area districts.[35]

Each author deftly handles their analysis of these policies and programs, making decades of segregation understandable to their respective readers. While they draw upon their academic backgrounds, Murphy and the Rothsteins generally write for nonacademic readers who seek ways to desegregate their communities, neighborhoods, and schools. They each note that their proposals will require commitment on the parts of activists, governments, and businesses, as well as realignment in the way people conceive of their lived environments and the role of government. The Rothsteins and Murphy successfully argue, however, that their proposals represent realistic steps for those committed to confronting and undoing the legacy of segregation. Their books draw upon history, political science, economics, and more. The Rothsteins note the danger of segregation, writing, "Once racial and class isolation becomes self-perpetuating it makes it even more difficult for us to come together, undermining our ability to forge a common national identity."[36] Murphy points to the hope in desegregating education, writing, "Every school could be dynamic and joyful if only adults would commit to building the proper foundation of anti-racism rather than racism; faith rather than fear; integration rather than segregation."[37] Murphy's and the Rothsteins' work complements the history of segregation, particularly as it exists after the Civil Rights era, while expanding beyond academic history into political activism. The way to desegregate and create a more just, equal, and flourishing society will not prove easy, but Murphy and the Rothsteins demonstrate the ways in which sociopolitical and economic systems maintain inequality and continue to do real and lasting harm into the twenty-first century. ■

1 "Justin Murphy," *Democrat and Chronicle*, accessed December 15, 2023, https://www.democratandchronicle.com/staff/2647405001/justin-murphy/.
2 "Richard Rothstein," Economic Policy Institute, accessed December 15, 2023, https://www.epi.org/people/richard-rothstein/; "Leah Rothstein," Economic Policy Institute, accessed December 15, 2023, https://www.epi.org/people/leah-rothstein/; "Leah Rothstein," HUD Exchange, accessed December 15, 2023, https://www.hudexchange.info/programs/nfhta/2023-fair-housing-conference/bios/leah-rothstein/.
3 Justin Murphy, *Your Children Are Very Greatly in Danger: School Segregation in Rochester, New York* (Ithaca, NY: Cornell University Press, 2022), 3.
4 Murphy, *Your Children*, 233.
5 Murphy, *Your Children*, 39.
6 Richard Rothstein and Leah Rothstein, *Just Action: How to Challenge Segregation Enacted Under the Color of Law* (New York: Liveright Publishing Corporation, 2023), 4.
7 Rothstein and Rothstein, *Just Action*, 5.
8 Thomas J. Sugrue, *Sweet Land of Liberty: The Forgotten Struggle for Civil Rights in the North* (New York: Random House, 2008), 303–4.
9 Sugrue, *Sweet Land of Liberty*, 201.
10 Sugrue, *Sweet Land of Liberty*, 204.

11 Lisa McGirr, *Suburban Warriors: The Origins of the New American Right* (Princeton, NJ: Princeton University Press, 2001), 43.
12 McGirr, *Suburban Warriors*, 53.
13 Matthew D. Lassiter, *The Silent Majority: Suburban Politics in the Sunbelt South* (Princeton, NJ: Princeton University Press, 2006), 4–6.
14 Lassiter, *The Silent Majority*, 53.
15 Lassiter, *The Silent Majority*, 148.
16 Lassiter, *The Silent Majority*, 198.
17 George Lipsitz, *The Possessive Investment in Whiteness: How White People Profit from Identity Politics*, Revised and Expanded Edition (Philadelphia, PA: Temple University Press, 2006), 18.
18 Murphy, *Your Children*, 28.
19 Murphy, *Your Children*, 39.
20 Murphy, *Your Children*, 59.
21 Murphy, *Your Children*, 75.
22 Murphy, *Your Children*, 82.
23 Murphy, *Your Children*, 103.
24 Murphy, *Your Children*, 157.
25 Rothstein and Rothstein, *Just Action*, 41.
26 Rothstein and Rothstein, *Just Action*, 65.
27 Rothstein and Rothstein, *Just Action*, 145.
28 Rothstein and Rothstein, *Just Action*, 47.
29 Rothstein and Rothstein, *Just Action*, 100.
30 Rothstein and Rothstein, *Just Action*, 112.
31 Rothstein and Rothstein, *Just Action*, 199.
32 Murphy, *Your Children*, 165.
33 Murphy, *Your Children*, 196.
34 Monroe County currently (ca. 2024) counts 21 distinct school districts.
35 Murphy, *Your Children*, 233–37.
36 Rothstein and Rothstein, *Just Action*, 84.
37 Murphy, *Your Children*, x.

BOOK REVIEW

New York's Burned-Over District: A Documentary History

edited by Spencer W. McBride and Jennifer Hull Dorsey.
Ithaca: Cornell University Press, 2023.

Erik R. Seeman, University at Buffalo

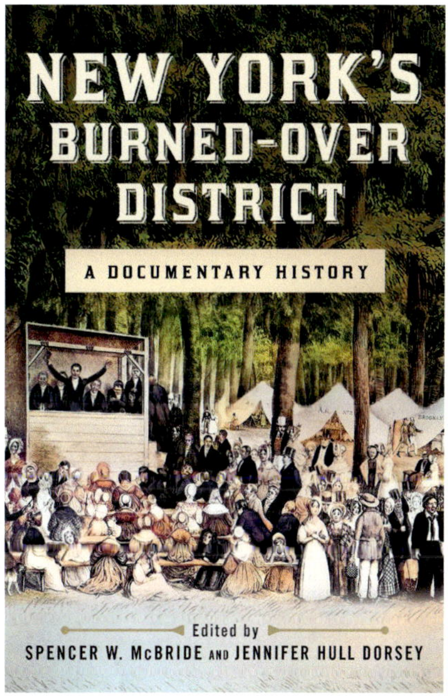

Nearly seventy-five years ago, Whitney R. Cross published *The Burned-Over District: The Social and Intellectual History of Enthusiastic Religion in Western New York, 1800–1850* (Ithaca, 1950), which is still cited by specialists. Indeed, the 2024 annual meeting of the Organization of American Historians featured an entire session devoted to the book. Part of the volume's longevity is owing simply to its resonant title, which conjures the intensity of the religious revivals that sped along the Erie Canal during the Second Great Awakening. More than that, though, Cross compellingly examines the social origins of the revivals among Yankee migrants, traces the expansion of Protestant denominations in the wake of preachers such as Charles Grandison Finney, and demonstrates connections between the revivals and the emergence of "ultraist" or radical reform. Even as several generations of scholars have added depth and texture to Cross's interpretations, no single book has yet supplanted it.

But now a new volume effectively complements it. Spencer W. McBride and Jennifer Hull Dorsey have compiled sixty-one documents that shed light on religion, politics, and reform in nineteenth-century New York. As they explain in the introduction, they have slightly expanded Cross's geographical and chronological reach. Whereas Cross defined his territory as New York west of the Catskills and Adirondacks, covering from 1800 to 1850, McBride and Dorsey add the Mohawk River Valley and encompass the years 1790 to 1860. These are small changes, but they allow the editors to include documents from Troy, Albany, and Watervliet, along with a few sources about Native Americans in the 1790s.

The editors have taken great care to ensure that nonspecialist readers can understand the documents. The volume begins with a helpful description of the editorial method and a brief introduction that situates the Burned-Over District both historically and historiographically. The documents are divided into eight "Parts," which are organized topically, but they also serve to move the story forward chronologically. Starting with a section on "Settlement," the parts include such topics as "Missionaries," "Revivals," "Intentional Communities," "Religion and New York Politics," and more. Best of all, not only does each part get its own introduction, but all sixty-one documents are prefaced by headnotes that explain who authored the document and why they wrote it. Readers will feel guided by expert hands through this collection.

Moreover, McBride and Dorsey have worked hard to avoid an overreliance on the "greatest hits": the best-known sources that have most shaped historical memory. Charles Finney gets his due, but he does not dominate the collection. Instead, the editors dig deeply into archives to find manuscript sources such as the wonderfully evocative missionary journal of Timothy Mather Cooley (1803) and the brief, but passionate, conversion narrative of Bradford King (1830). The collection includes sources about the wide range of new religious movements that jostled for attention in the Burned-Over District: Shakers, Mormons, Millerites, and more. The volume also includes a greater diversity of sources than one finds in Cross. Whereas Cross relies on documents written almost exclusively by Anglo-American men, McBride and Dorsey feature sources by women (including a letter from the Grimké sisters), African Americans (such as Samuel Ringgold Ward's breathtaking account of his time as pastor to an all-white church east of Rochester), and Native Americans (including an 1805 speech by the Seneca leader Sagoyewatha [or Red Jacket]).

Undergraduate and graduate students comprise the audience that will likely benefit most from this collection. One can imagine an instructor organizing a course around the volume, assigning one section per week along with relevant secondary readings and leaving several weeks at the end for independent research. But realistically, such courses will be rare. Instead, more instructors will recommend the volume to students writing senior theses or master's theses. It's a great place for them to start their research. Members of the reading public might pick up the volume, but only those most passionate about the topic will be able to push through nearly 400 pages of nineteenth-century prose.

Scholars will wonder whether the introduction or the selection of documents offer a novel argument. Not really, though two things struck me: First, the sources were less dramatic than I expected. As the editors put it, "If we look to the way many of the residents of the Burned-over District described the several waves of religious enthusiasm that swept the area, we catch a softer and less fiery view of the district."[1] This is borne out throughout the volume, but especially in the section on "Church Development," which features church constitutions, trustee reports, and accounts of donations. These sources demonstrate the "pragmatic—even mundane—work required of church members" to build and sustain their denominations.[2] It's a useful reminder that the "Burned-over" sobriquet offers a partial view of a period that, after all, lasted half a century. The swooning and crying that marked camp meetings did not characterize the daily experience of religion in antebellum New York.

Second, the volume sparked an epiphany of sorts: A collection of documents is necessarily shaggier than a monograph. When writing a monograph, a skilled historian selects examples and quotations that support an argument, thereby stripping away some of the complexity of how people lived their lives. A documentary collection—especially one as ecumenical as this in its inclusion of diverse voices—is messier and more comprehensive, and therefore probably a better representation of the time and place in question. In their wide-ranging search for documents to represent the Burned-Over District in all its complexity, McBride and Dorsey have crafted a worthy complement to Cross's classic. ■

1 McBride and Hull Dorsey, 10.
2 McBride and Hull Dorsey, 160.

The Hill Cumorah Legacy Project: Capturing Rochester's Latter-Day Saint History

Daniel Gorman Jr.

When you think of the world's major religious sites, you may not think of Rochester, New York. If you drive forty-five minutes east of the city, however, you'll reach Palmyra, New York, a town with holy sites in abundance. Members of the Church of Jesus Christ of Latter-Day Saints (Mormons) believe that the prophet Joseph Smith Jr. received visions in the woods known as the Sacred Grove and recovered the golden plates of the Book of Mormon from the Hill Cumorah. The modern Book of Mormon was first published in Palmyra. To Mormons, Palmyra is where God restored communication with humanity, and Greater Rochester is where Smith launched a church.

The LDS Church celebrated Palmyra's religious history by staging an outdoor play, the Hill Cumorah Pageant, every July from 1937 to 2019 (save for a few years during World War II). Intended as a missionary tool, the Pageant reenacted key stories from the Book of Mormon for the public. Over time, LDS families joined the cast and crew alongside the missionaries. Interest grew to the point that applications were needed to choose participants. By the 1980s, Pageant season was a fusion of pilgrimage, summer stock theater, and sleepaway camp for many Latter-Day Saints, who sustained the nineteenth-century tradition of grand community pageants.

I first saw the Pageant in 2017 and was blown away by its scale. Afterward, I wrote about the Pageant for *Sacred Matters Magazine*, and I saw the 2018 and 2019 productions, but grad-school commitments prevented me from studying the show further.[1] Meanwhile, the Church announced a shift away from pageants to other, more portable forms of missionary work. The Pageant was expensive, and the number of non-LDS viewers—the people whom missionaries hoped to reach—was declining. The final Pageant was scheduled for 2020. Then COVID hit. The show was delayed until 2021, then canceled altogether.

In 2021, Tamar Carroll, the chair of the Department of History at Rochester Institute of Technology, recruited me to teach "Digital History" for the spring 2022 semester. The course would introduce students to the potential of digital technology—mapping, scanning, digital storytelling, audio recording, et cetera—for historical research. Students would produce a collaborative project by semester's end. I saw the course as an opportunity to preserve the history of the Hill Cumorah Pageant while memories of it were fresh in the minds of Rochester residents.

With Dr. Carroll's support, I contacted several Rochester-area Church leaders and pitched the Hill Cumorah Legacy

Project. For their practicum, RIT students would catalog Pageant artifacts sourced from the community (an activity known as a "History Harvest"), record oral-history interviews with Pageant alumni, and transcribe the interviews for accessibility.[2] The Church representatives were pleasantly surprised, I think, by the project, which would see mostly non-LDS students interview Saints about closely held matters of religion. Specifically, the Church officials were intrigued by the idea of collecting Pageant mementos from community members. After the meeting, the officials introduced me to LDS Church archivist Elizabeth Heath, who said that the students' work could be preserved with the Church History Department in Utah.

In my experience, digital history courses tend to emphasize the digital *or* the history. You either learn about technology at the expense of historical content, or you learn about history at the expense of technology. I wanted to give students a decent amount of both topics—the technical skills that they needed for their assignments *and* enough LDS history to conduct meaningful interviews. To achieve this goal, I often alternated between "digital" and "history" class days. This pattern made the course feel choppy at times.

Other issues arose. According to the end-of-semester survey, one student disliked that the course project's topic was chosen in advance, feeling that religion didn't belong in a digital history course. Another respondent wrote that producing two digital projects during the semester instead of one would have inspired more student interest. During class discussions, students expressed that they weren't accustomed to discussing religion. The prospect of contacting strangers to schedule interviews caused some anxiety. The most challenging situation was when one student refused to interview Pageant alumni because of personal grievances with the LDS Church. In the end, I let that student complete an alternative oral history assignment.

That student was an outlier, though. Most students said that they enjoyed their conversations with Pageant alumni, who shared their stories at length and with enthusiasm. Students were excited that both RIT and the Church History Department would preserve their work; it would not disappear after the semester. Furthermore, students enjoyed our in-class "History Harvest," in which we photographed and catalogued Pageant artifacts from the private collection of Gerry and Gail Argetsinger. Gerry is a former Pageant director and Gail a former Pageant costume designer. Their collection consists mainly of costumes, but it also includes photos, stage props, documents, and memorabilia. Students had fun laying the costumes out on desks and looking for the best camera angles to capture their intricate details.

Unfortunately, there wasn't enough time in the semester to assemble the website fully. The course ended, and students could not yet list the finished site on their resumes. It took well into 2023 to secure copyright clearance from the LDS Church to publish the Argetsinger collection online, since every item made for the Pageant technically was made under Church auspices. Nevertheless, by fall 2023, the bulk of the students' work was online. Any items that lacked copyright clearance were still saved internally at RIT and the Church History Department. The RIT Libraries and the Department of History are committed to supporting the project website. In summer 2023, student intern Emmarose Tabin worked with faculty and library staff to migrate the project to the latest version of the Omeka content-management system.

The updated project is available at https://www.hillcumorahlegacy.net/.

It is my hope that the Hill Cumorah Legacy Project will inspire more research into Western New York's LDS history. Much has been written about Joseph Smith and the migration of the Church from New York to Utah, but less has been written about the rebuilding of Rochester's LDS community in the 1900s. The History Harvest approach is promising. Who knows what records of Church activities are sitting in the attics of Rochesterians? Another avenue for research is local newspaper coverage of Mormon topics. Researchers could consult the free NYS Historic Newspapers database or the microfilmed newspaper collections at the Rochester Public Library.

With any luck, the Hill Cumorah Legacy Project will be the first of many collaborations between Rochester's Latter-Day Saints, historians, and history students. ■

1 Daniel Gorman Jr., "The Center of the Mormon World: The Hill Cumorah Pageant," *Sacred Matters Magazine* (Aug. 30, 2017), https://sacredmattersmagazine.com/the-center-of-the-mormon-world-the-hill-cumorah-pageant/.

2 See Patrick D. Jones and William G. Thomas, III, *History Harvest*, University of Nebraska–Lincoln, accessed Jan. 12, 2024, https://historyharvest.unl.edu/, Creative Commons License (CC BY 4.0), https://creativecommons.org/licenses/by/4.0/.

HIST 326: Digital History (3 units)

Tuesday/Thursday 11 Am–12:15 PM,
George Eastman Hall (EAS)-3355, Spring 2022
Rochester Institute of Technology

Instructor: Daniel Gorman Jr. (he/his/him)
History PhD Candidate, University of Rochester
Virtual Office Hours: Wednesdays 10–11:30
Additional office hours by appointment.
Course Librarians: Rebekah Walker and Cami Goldowitz

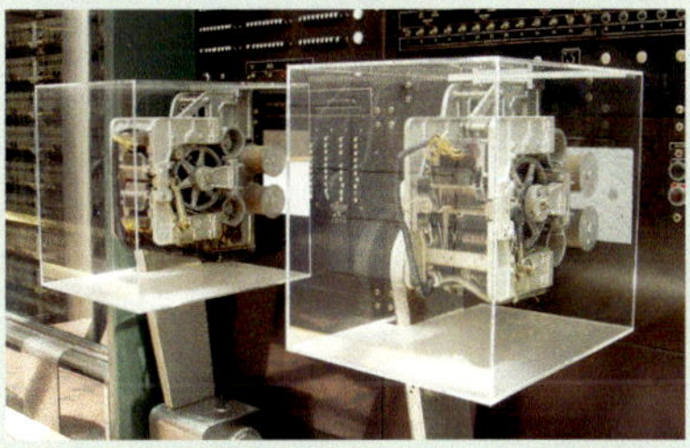

Photo Credit: Daderot [pseud.], "Harvard-IBM Mark I Computer, detail of Input/Output and control" (July 2005), Wikimedia Commons, last modified March 24, 2007, CC BY-SA 3.0, https://commons.wikimedia.org/wiki/File:Harvard_Mark_I_Computer_-_Input-Output_Details.jpg.

This course is an introduction to the theory, methods, and applications of digital history. Digital history is **the use of computer, audiovisual, and mobile device technology to produce and share knowledge of the past**. The course has three primary components. The first component is learning about **the development of digital history**, key concepts and practices, and questions of diversity, equity, and inclusion in digital projects. The second component is **technology demonstrations**, showing how digital technologies can be used for history research and education. The third component is a **practicum in digital history**. Our focus is preserving local religious history. We will build a web exhibit about the Hill Cumorah Pageant, an annual theatrical production that the Church of Jesus Christ of Latter-day Saints hosted outside of Rochester from 1937 to 2019. To do so, we will collaborate with community stakeholders and learn about Rochester's connections to Joseph Smith and the Mormon tradition. The project will be hosted online at https://cumorahlegacy.omeka.net/.

By the end of this class, students will:

- Have a working knowledge of the theories, methods, and best practices of digital history.
- Contribute to a public-facing digital history project.
- Learn about project management and community engagement.
- Have a greater understanding of Western New York's religious history.

What are your goals for the course? Write them here.

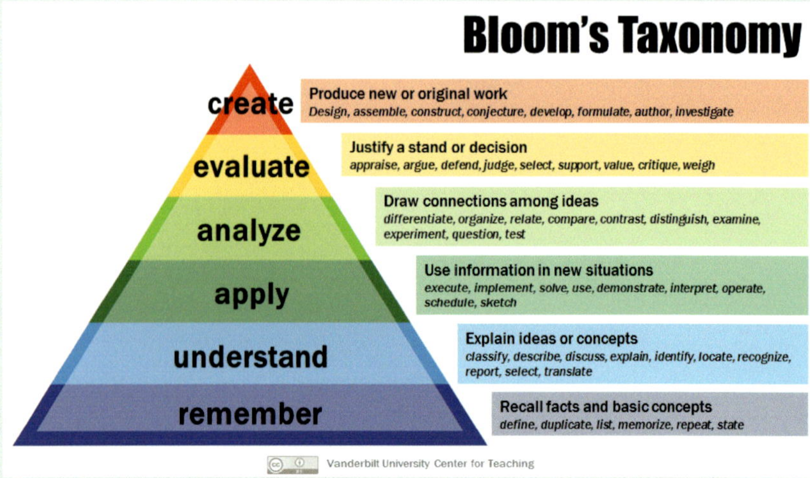

Source: Vanderbilt University Center for Teaching, acc. Apr. 30, 2018, https://www.flickr.com/photos/vandycft/29428436431, CC-BY-2.0.

Course Format and Technical Requirements

This course is a seminar. I will give lectures, but much of class will consist of discussions, tech demonstrations, and collaborative work on projects. An Internet-enabled computer or tablet is required for this course. It is your responsibility to stay focused and not get distracted online! Please do not use your cell phone in class unless you are instructed to do so or if you use your phone for an accessibility accommodation.

During this course, you will submit written assignments through MyCourses. Two digital history assignments, which I discuss below, will be submitted through Omeka and RIT's Google Drive. Your digital history projects will ultimately go on the publicly available website https://cumorahlegacy.omeka.net/ and remain there after the course ends. **If you do not wish to make your projects public, please let me know via email by Tuesday, February 8**.

In the event of a University-wide emergency (e.g., a pandemic closure, a weather disaster, or other crisis), course requirements, classes, deadlines and grading schemes are subject to change. Course changes may include alternative delivery methods, alternative methods of interaction with the instructor and/or classmates, new course materials, a revised attendance policy, a revised semester calendar, and/or an adjusted grading scheme.

Any emergency updates to the course, including COVID-19 updates, will be shared by email and posted on MyCourses.

Intellectual Honesty

As an institution of higher learning, RIT expects students to behave honestly and ethically at all times, especially when submitting work for evaluation in conjunction with any course or degree requirement. The Department of History encourages all students to be familiar with the RIT Honor Code (https://www.rit.edu/academicaffairs/policiesmanual/p030) and the RIT Student Academic Integrity Policy (https://www.rit.edu/academicaffairs/policiesmanual/d080).

You are encouraged to discuss course readings with other students, and you'll work on collaborative projects. **Papers and reports, however, must be written independently**. Unacceptable actions include plagiarism (copying others' words and/or failing to cite all of your sources), submitting past assignments, and the falsification of data.

Certain materials used in this course are protected by copyright and may not be copied or distributed by students. You can find more information at http://www.rit.edu/academicaffairs/policiesmanual/sectionC/C3_2.html. When sharing copyrighted content on the Internet with your classmates, please make sure that you link to a legal source. Repeated access to illegal sources may cause you or your classmates to receive warnings through the Copyright Alert System as well as possible downgrades in Internet service.

To gain appropriate help for your papers, I encourage you to consult the University Writing Program.

Accommodation Statement

RIT is committed to providing academic adjustments to students with disabilities. If you would like to request academic adjustments such as testing modifications due to a disability, please contact the Disability Services Office. Contact information for the DSO and information about how to request adjustments can be found at www.rit.edu/dso. After you receive academic adjustment approval, it is imperative that you contact me as early as possible so that we can work out whatever arrangement is necessary.

The Disability Services Office is located in Student Alumni Union 1150, can be contacted by telephone at 585-475-2023, can be contacted by email at dso@rit.edu, and offers further information at https://www.rit.edu/disabilityservices/who-we-support. The director of Disability Services is Catherine Lewis. The Test Center coordinator is Alyson Jones. The assistant director is Shelley Zoeke.

Religious Holidays: Should you have a religious observance during the semester, please notify me and we can make arrangements for you to make up any missed work.

Safe Space Policy, Title IX Policy, and Student Resources

I believe in the importance of campus safe zones, where students feel free to ask any question on their minds, and where they feel respected, valued, and welcomed. You are invited to share the name you want to be called and the pronouns you want others to use. When we discuss controversial topics in class, I will give you advance warning of sensitive material. **I will not accept discrimination of any form in my classroom.**

Title IX violations are taken very seriously at RIT. RIT is committed to investigating complaints of sexual discrimination, sexual harassment, sexual assault, and other sexual misconduct, and to ensuring that appropriate action is taken to stop the behavior, prevent its recurrence, and remedy its effects. Please view the Title IX Rights & Resources (https://www.rit.edu/fa/compliance/title-ix) at RIT.

This course participates in the RIT Starfish academic alert system, which is designed to promote student success through communication between students, instructors, and advisors. When I am concerned about a student's academic performance, I may raise an academic alert to notify the student as well as their advisor(s). If you receive an academic alert email, it is your responsibility to contact me ASAP to discuss the issue and identify resources to help move you forward. For more information about the Starfish system, visit www.rit.edu/starfish.

Academic stress is an unavoidable part of the college experience, and it can be compounded by unexpected setbacks, life changes, or other events outside the classroom. **Please take care of yourself throughout the term**. If you have a personal issue pressing upon you, I am available to connect you to relevant campus resources. I am not a confidential resource, but I can help you connect with a confidential resource. I also encourage you to speak with your academic advisor. Additionally, to help you navigate any issues that may arise, the following resources are available to RIT students:

- Academic Success Center: https://www.rit.edu/academicsuccesscenter/.
- Access Services: https://www.rit.edu/ntid/das.
- COVID-19 Resources—RIT Ready: https://www.rit.edu/ready/.
- Counseling and Psychological Services: https://www.rit.edu/counseling/get-support.
- Deaf and Hard-of-Hearing Student Support: https://www.rit.edu/ntid/support-services/other-colleges.
- Disability Services Office: https://www.rit.edu/disabilityservices/.
- Diversity and Inclusion Resources: https://www.rit.edu/diversity/.
- Process for Emergency Closing (weather, etc.): https://finweb.rit.edu/grms/close_university_process.html.
- Emergency Preparedness: http://finweb.rit.edu/publicsafety/preparedness/.
- FoodShare: https://campusgroups.rit.edu/foodshare/rit-foodshare-pre-packaged-grocery-bag-request-program/.
- Future Stewards Program: https://www.rit.edu/diversity/futurestewards.
- Information & Technology Services: https://www.rit.edu/its/. Help line: 585-475-5000.
- Libraries: http://library.rit.edu/.
- Multicultural Center for Academic Success: https://www.rit.edu/diversity/multicultural-center-academic-success-mcas.
- MyCourses Support: https://www.rit.edu/academicaffairs/tls/course-delivery/academic-technology/mycourses, https://www.rit.edu/academicaffairs/tls/quick-help.
- Ombuds Office: https://www.rit.edu/ombuds/.
- Policy Prohibiting Discrimination, Harassment, and Retaliation: https://www.rit.edu/academicaffairs/policiesmanual/c060.

- Public Safety: https://www.rit.edu/fa/publicsafety/.
- The Q Center (LGBTQ student support): https://campusgroups.rit.edu/qcenter/home/.
- *Report an Incident* (COVID Protocol Violations, Concerns about a Student, Crime or Policy Violation, Title IX Concern, Ethics and Compliance, *or* Biased-Related Incident): https://www.rit.edu/reporting-incident.
    - Direct Link for Ethics and Compliance Reporting: https://secure.ethicspoint.com/domain/media/en/gui/11003/index.html.
    - Direct Link for Title IX Sexual Harassment, Discrimination and Sexual Misconduct Reporting: https://cm.maxient.com/reportingform.php?RochesterInstofTech&layout_id=25.
- Spirituality & Religious Life: https://www.rit.edu/studentaffairs/religion/.
- Student Health Center: https://www.rit.edu/studenthealth/.
- Teaching & Learning Services: https://www.rit.edu/academicaffairs/tls/. Email: tlsupport@rit.edu. Help Line: 585-438-5219.
- Title IX Rights & Resources: https://www.rit.edu/fa/compliance/title-ix.
- University Writing Program: https://www.rit.edu/writing/.
- Zoom Support: https://rit.zoom.us/.

Course Assignments and Grading

We have one textbook for this course that is available in the RIT Barnes & Noble: Matthew Bowman, *The Mormon People: The Making of an American Faith***.** New York: Random House, 2012, ISBN: 9780812983364. It is also available as an e-book from Wallace Library. All other homework readings will be available through MyCourses or freely available on the Internet.

If you want to learn more about digital humanities technology, I recommend the free resources available from *The Programming Historian* (https://programminghistorian.org/en/lessons/) and DARIAH (https://teach.dariah.eu/). Relevant courses are available through LinkedIn Learning, Coursera, EdX, Udemy, StackSkills, and Library Juice Academy. RIT has a LinkedIn Learning subscription (https://infoguides.rit.edu/linkedinlearning). You often must pay for the other sites' content.

Assignments:

- All assignments, including participation, will be graded on a 100-point scale.
- All written assignments will be submitted via MyCourses.
- Digital projects will be submitted through Omeka and Google Drive (see details below).
- We are living through a global pandemic. We've been through a lot in the past two years. Every student has the right to **one absence, no explanation required**, AND **one day off from doing the homework, no explanation required**.
- Late assignments will lose 1/3 of a letter grade for *each day* that they are not submitted. **This means that you technically have a 24-hour grace period to submit all assignments without losing points**. If you need more time because of pandemic-related problems, let me know, and I will support extensions when possible. (It gets challenging near the end of the semester.)

■ If you use your absence/no-homework privilege on the day that an assignment is due, then your assignment will be due at the same time on the next day.

■ With the exception of medical leave scenarios, **you will not pass the course with five or more absences**.

(1) **Digital history report (10% of semester grade)**: You will write a 750-word report about a history website or podcast that you will select from a pre-circulated list.
(2) **Oregon Trail response paper (10% of semester grade)**: This short assignment will ask you to play the classic video game and write a 750-word reflection about the experience.
(3) **Omeka item cataloguing project (10% of semester grade)**: Using a smartphone camera or a digital camera, you will produce digital images of a primary source/artifact related to the Hill Cumorah Pageant. You will upload your object as an "item" in Omeka and provide metadata and a description for it.
(4) **Oral history project (35% of semester grade)**: Working in pairs (or trios, if necessary), you will interview a past participant in the Hill Cumorah Pageant. The project will consist of three parts:

- ■ (A) An initial **list of questions** for your interview subject that you submit to me for review, worth 10% of your semester grade.
- ■ (B) An **audio recording** of the interview, saved in MP3, M4A/AAC, or WAV format, worth 15% of your semester grade.
- ■ (C) A **transcript** of the interview, saved in .docx format, worth 10% of your semester grade.

Note: Both students in each pair will receive the same grade—unless it comes to my attention that one person did not contribute. In that case, the student who did the work will receive the grade, and the other student will receive an automatic failing grade on the project.
(5) **"Behind the scenes" paper reflecting on your scanning and oral history projects (10% of semester grade)**: This 1,000-word paper is intended to be a reflection on your scanning and oral history projects. Describe your experience of working on these projects. What technologies (hardware and software) did you use? Did you encounter any technical problems? What, if anything, would you do differently on a future digital history project? Finally, what did you learn about producing historical materials for the general public?
(6) **Three textbook quizzes (15% of final grade, or 5% each)**: You will complete these open-book quizzes via MyCourses outside of class.
(7) **Class participation (10% of final grade)**: As this course is a seminar, participation is essential. Your participation grade will be based on regular class attendance, active participation in discussions, and your contributions to in-class projects and activities.

If you quote or paraphrase material from a website, video, course reading, or other source in your writing assignments, you must cite it with footnotes or endnotes and a "Works Cited" section, following the Chicago Manual of Style, 17th edition. The Chicago Manual is accessible via the RIT Libraries catalog: https://albert.rit.edu/record=b2778109~S3.

I use the following grade scheme:
A: 93–100%. **A-**: 90–92.99%. **B+**: 87–89.99%. **B**: 83–86.99%. **B-**: 80–82.99%. **C+**: 77–79.99%. **C**: 73–76.99%. **C-**: 70–72.99%. **D**: 65–69.99%. **F**: Failure (64.99% or below).

About Collaboration: Working on a team-based, collaborative project may be a change from history classes you took previously. Group work can be stressful at times. If you are unclear about your role in the group or worry that you are being asked to do too much, please see me immediately.

Calendar of Classes and Assignments

Week 1: Course Introduction

Tuesday, January 11: Welcome to HIST 326

- Opening conversation about digital history.
- Watch in class: Primers on the Hill Cumorah Project:
    - News 8 WROC, "Hill Cumorah Pageant in Palmyra to end in 2020," Oct. 28, 2018, https://www.youtube.com/watch?v=mKk3G463Aq4. (Update: This Pageant was canceled; 2019 was the last year it was held.)
    - Curtis Whitear and Radiowest, "A Mormon Pageant: The Hill Cumorah," uploaded Feb. 29, 2019, https://www.youtube.com/watch?v=KNrFov_3L2s.
- Syllabus review.

Thursday, January 13: The History of Digital History

Read before class:

- Susan Hockey, "The History of Humanities Computing," *A Companion to Digital Humanities* (Oxford: Blackwell, 2004), http://www.digitalhumanities.org/companion/view?docId=blackwell/9781405103213/9781405103213.xml&chunk.id=ss1-2-1. Approx. 10 pages.
- Douglas Seefeldt and William G. Thomas, III, "What is Digital History? A Look at Some Exemplar Projects," Faculty Publications, Paper 98, Univ. of Nebraska Lincoln, 2009, https://digitalcommons.unl.edu/historyfacpub/98/. 8 pages.

In class:

We'll look at some early digital history projects (and some throwback links for fun):

- Father Busa and the *Index Thomisticus*: https://www.corpusthomisticum.org/it/index.age.
- *Women Writers Project*: https://www.wwp.northeastern.edu/.
- *Rosetti Archive*: http://www.rossettiarchive.org/.
- *The William Blake Archive*: http://www.blakearchive.org/.
- Original *Space Jam* website (1996): https://www.spacejam.com/1996/.
- Library of Congress *American Memory*: https://memory.loc.gov/ammem/index.html.

To show the old interface, I may use archived pages from the Internet Archive.

- *Valley of the Shadow Project*: https://valley.lib.virginia.edu/.
- Steven Mintz's *Digital History* (U.S. history) site: http://www.digitalhistory.uh.edu/.
- "Snowfall," *New York Times*, 2012: https://www.nytimes.com/projects/2012/snow-fall/index.html#/?part=tunnel-creek.

Week 2: Digital Projects and Mormon History

Monday, January 17, 2022: Martin Luther King Jr. Day. There is no class today, but I encourage you to attend the campus-wide celebration!

Tuesday, January 18: Approaches to Digital History

Read before class:

- Roy Rosenzweig and Daniel J. Cohen, *Digital History* (2006), "Exploring the History Web," https://chnm.gmu.edu/digitalhistory/exploring/. Approx. 27 pages.
- Stephen Robertson, "The Differences between Digital Humanities and Digital History," *Debates in the Digital Humanities 2016*, https://dhdebates.gc.cuny.edu/read/untitled/section/ed4a1145-7044-42e9-a898-5ff8691b6628#ch25. 8 pages.

In class:

- "Best Practices for Digital Humanities Projects," University of Nebraska Lincoln: https://cdrh.unl.edu/articles/best_practices.
- Discussion about history podcasts.
- Untranscribed podcasts:
    - *Ben Franklin's World*: https://benfranklinsworld.com/episode-transcriptions/.
- Transcribed podcasts:
    - *In Geveb*: https://ingeveb.org/tags/podcast.
    - *The Religious Studies Project*: https://www.religiousstudiesproject.com/.
    - *Sawbones*: https://maximumfun.org/podcasts/sawbones/?_post-type=transcript.
    - StoryCorps introduction video by David Isay, YouTube, Sept. 15, 2015: https://youtu.be/KGCD1XR0WPk.

Thursday, January 20: Introduction to Mormon History

Read before class:

- Matthew Bowman, *The Mormon People* (2012), Introduction and Chapters 1–3. 102 pages total.

Complete before class begins:

- MyCourses quiz on *The Mormon People*, Chapters 1–3.

In class:

- Discussion of Rochester's Mormon history and our study of the Hill Cumorah Pageant.
- "Timeline: Prominent Religious Events and People in American History," Association of Religion Data Archives (ARDA), https://www.thearda.com/timeline/tlRank1to2.asp.

- LDS Church's *Church History* website: https://history.churchofjesuschrist.org/.
- Dale Broadhurst, *Uncle Dale's Readings in Early Mormon History*: www.sidneyrigdon.com/dbroadhu/artindex.htm.

Week 3: Diversity, Equity, and Inclusion in Digital History

Tuesday, January 25: Gender and Race in Digital Humanities Projects

Read **two** of these articles before class:

- Kimberly Christen, "Does Information Really Want to be Free? Indigenous Knowledge Systems and the Question of Openness," *International Journal of Communications* 6 (2012): 2870–93, https://ijoc.org/index.php/ijoc/article/view/1618/828.
- Catherine D'Ignazio and Lauren F. Klein, *Data Feminism* (MIT Press, 2020), Chapter 2, "Collect, Analyze, Imagine, Teach," https://data-feminism.mitpress.mit.edu/pub/ei7cogfn/release/2. Approx. 38 pages.
- Melissa Dinsman, "The Digital in the Humanities: An Interview with Jessica Marie Johnson," *LA Review of Books*, July 23, 2016, https://lareviewofbooks.org/article/digital-humanities-interview-jessica-marie-johnson/. Approx. 15 pages.

In class: Projects and Platforms:

- "Black Digital Humanities Projects & Resources" (index): bit.ly/Black-DH-List.
- *Colored Conventions Project*: https://coloredconventions.org/.
- *Click! The Ongoing Feminist Revolution*: https://www.cliohistory.org/click/.
- Digital Library of the Caribbean: https://www.dloc.com/.
- Mukurtu: https://mukurtu.org/.
- Mukurtu Examples:
    - Huna Heritage Digital Archives: http://archives.hunaheritage.org/.
    - Plateau Peoples' Web Portal, "Statement of Commitment": https://plateauportal.libraries.wsu.edu/about.
    - Passamaquoddy People: https://passamaquoddypeople.com.
- *The Quilt Index*: https://quiltindex.org/.
- Script Encoding Initiative: https://linguistics.berkeley.edu/sei/.
- *South Asian American Digital Archive*: https://www.saada.org.
- Traditional Knowledge Labels: https://localcontexts.org/labels/traditional-knowledge-labels/.
- *The Willa Cather Archive*: https://cather.unl.edu/.

Thursday, January 27: Mormon History Part II

Read before class:

- Bowman, *The Mormon People*, Chapters 4–6, pages 96–183.

Complete before class begins:

- MyCourses quiz on *The Mormon People*, Chapters 4–6.

In class:

- Class visit by Brighton, NY, LDS Bishop Brian Surprenant.
- Discussion of Mormon history.

Week 4: Project Management

Tuesday, February 1: Thinking about Project Management

Read before class:

- Miriam Posner, "How Did They Make That?" August 29, 2013, http://miriamposner.com/blog/how-did-they-make-that/. Approx. 9 pages.
- Mary Rizzo, "Every tool is a weapon: Why the digital humanities movement needs public history," 2012, https://ncph.org/history-at-work/every-tool-is-a-weapon/. 3 pages.
- "Agile Project Management: A Comprehensive Guide" (Kanbanize): https://kanbanize.com/agile/project-management. Approx. 14 pages.
- **Skim**: *Project Management for the Digital Humanities* (Emory Center for Digital Scholarship): https://scholarblogs.emory.edu/pm4dh/.

In class:

- "Digital Humanities and the Seward Family Digital Archive" (University of Rochester YouTube channel): https://www.youtube.com/watch?v=YNs2jhuPspw.
- *The History Harvest*: https://historyharvest.unl.edu/about.
- Seward Project, "Building a Digital Collection": https://www.youtube.com/watch?v=VgYyqhcjNV8.

Thursday, February 3: Content Management Systems / Introduction to Omeka

Read before class:

- Review the website for the Omeka app: https://omeka.org/.
- National Council on Public History Code of Ethics and Professional Conduct: https://ncph.org/about/governance-committees/code-of-ethics-and-professional-conduct/. Approx. 4 pages.

In class:

- Omeka workshop with Rebekah Walker.
- Creating Metadata with the Dublin Core Metadata Initiative: https://dublincore.org/resources/userguide/creating_metadata/.

Week 5: Starting the Hill Cumorah Legacy Project

Tuesday, February 8: Mormon History Wrap-Up / Turning to the Hill Cumorah Pageant

Read before class:

- Watch the official recording of the Hill Cumorah Pageant: https://www.churchofjesuschrist.org/media/video/2021-06-1000-hill-cumorah-pageant?lang=eng.

■ Bowman, *The Mormon People*, Chapters 7–8 and Conclusion, pages 184–262.
■ Megan Sanborn Jones, *Contemporary Mormon Pageantry: Seeking after the Dead* (2018), Chapter 1, "The Past is Never Dead." Posted in MyCourses.

Complete before class begins:
■ MyCourses quiz on *The Mormon People*, Chapters 7–Conclusion.

In class:
■ Visit by former Pageant director Jerry Argetsinger.
■ Discussion of the Hill Cumorah Pageant's history and operations.

Thursday, February 10: Introduction to Oral History
Read before class in this recommended order:
■ "Introduction to Oral History," Baylor University Institute for Oral History: https://www.baylor.edu/content/services/document.php/43912.pdf. 21 pages.
■ "Oral History Association Statement on Ethics": https://www.oralhistory.org/oha-statement-on-ethics/. 3 pages.
■ "Archiving Oral History": https://www.oralhistory.org/archives-principles-and-best-practices-overview/. 4 pages.

In class:
■ Discussion of oral history concepts and methods.
■ Assigning interview subjects for the Hill Cumorah Legacy Project.
■ Atomic Heritage Foundation's Voices of the Manhattan Project: https://www.manhattanprojectvoices.org.
■ Studs Terkel Radio Archive: https://studsterkel.wfmt.com.
■ University of Kentucky Louie B. Nunn Center for Oral History: https://libraries.uky.edu/libpage.php?lweb_id=11&llib_id=13.

Week 6: Oral History / Virtual Reality

Tuesday, February 15: Drafting Oral History Questions
Read before class:
■ "Best Practices": https://www.oralhistory.org/best-practices/. 4 pages.
■ "For Participants in Oral History Interviews": https://www.oralhistory.org/for-participants-in-oral-history-interviews/. 3 pages.

In class:
■ Review of how to conduct oral history interviews.
■ Working in pairs, you will prepare questions for the person you will interview.

Thursday, February 17: 3D Models and History

Read before class:

- Bob Marcotte, "How do you bring a castle home with you?" University of Rochester Newscenter, Dec. 3, 2019, https://www.rochester.edu/newscenter/virtual-tour-elmina-castle-409602/. 5 pages.
- Sifan Ye, Michael Jarvis, Ting Wu, and Yuhao Zhu, "Digital Reconstruction of Elmina Castle for Mobile Virtual Reality via Point-based Detail Transfer," preprint, 2020–21, https://arxiv.org/pdf/2012.10739.pdf. 9 pages.

Due by the start of class (11 AM ET): Your group's list of oral history questions.

- Please submit your list of oral history questions as a Word, plain text, or Pages file via MyCourses.

In class:

- *Chronoleap*: https://chronopoints.eecs.ucf.edu/portfolio_page/chronoleap/.
- *Digital Elmina*: https://digitalelmina.org/.
- *Digital Karnark*: https://humtech.ucla.edu/project/digital-karnak/.
- *Paris 3D*: https://www.3ds.com/stories/paris-3d/.
- *Resurrect 3D*: https://www.library.rochester.edu/spaces/studio-x/resources/resurrect3d.
- *Rome Reborn*: https://www.romereborn.org/.
- *The Zamani Project*: https://zamaniproject.org/data-types.html.

Week 7: Project Development

Tuesday, February 22: Workshop: Imaging Objects from the Hill Cumorah Pageant

Read before class:

- None. Work on your digital history report.

Due by the start of class (11 AM ET): Digital history report.

In class:

- Visit by Jerry Argetsinger.
- We will scan and photograph artifacts and primary sources, courtesy of the Jerry and Gail Argetsinger Collection, for the Hill Cumorah Project.

Scanning apps that offer alternatives to a basic cell phone camera:

- PhotoScan by Google: https://www.google.com/photos/scan/.
- iPhone scanning apps: Prizmo (https://creaceed.com/iprizmo), Scanner Pro (https://readdle.com/scannerpro), and Genius Scan (https://apps.apple.com/us/app/genius-scan-pdf-scanner/id377672876).
- Android scanning app: CamScanner (https://play.google.com/store/apps/details?id=com.intsig.camscanner).

Thursday, February 24: Introduction to Metadata and Library Science

Read before class:

■ Denise D. Meringolo, "Civic Engagement," *The Inclusive Historian's Handbook*, May 23, 2019, https://inclusivehistorian.com/civic-engagement/. Approx. 6 pages.

■ Rosenzweig and Cohen, *Digital History*, "Owning the Past?" https://chnm.gmu.edu/digitalhistory/copyright/. Approx. 38 pages.

In class:

■ Creative Commons Licenses: https://creativecommons.org/.

■ AV Preserve "Cost of Inaction Calculator": https://coi.weareavp.com/.

■ CESSDA SaW Archive Development Canvas: https://zenodo.org/record/3662469.

■ Digitization Cost Calculator: https://dashboard.diglib.org/.

■ The Internet Archive: https://archive.org.

■ Clips from "Internet Archive 25th Anniversary," YouTube livestream, Oct. 21, 2021: https://youtu.be/pzMlOtrhEwc.

■ Permanent.org: https://www.permanent.org/.

Week 8: Maps and Consoles

Tuesday, March 1: Digital Maps and Geographic Information Systems

Read before class:

■ Stephen Robertson, "Putting Harlem on the Map," *Writing History in the Digital Age* (2013), https://quod.lib.umich.edu/d/dh/12230987.0001.001/1:8/--writing-history-in-the-digital-age?g=dculture;rgn=div1;view=fulltext;xc=1#8.2. Approx. 9 pages.

■ Explore any **two** of the following spatial history sites:

- ■ Curatescape Projects: https://curatescape.org/projects/.
- ■ HyperCities: http://www.hypercities.com/.
- ■ *PhilaPlace*: http://www.philaplace.org/.
- ■ Philly History: https://www.phillyhistory.org/PhotoArchive/Home.aspx.
- ■ Social Explorer: https://www.socialexplorer.com/.
- ■ *Spatial History Project*: https://web.stanford.edu/group/spatialhistory/cgi-bin/site/index.php.

In class:

■ ArcGIS Workshop with Blair Tinker from the University of Rochester.

Thursday, March 3: Video Games and History

Read before class:

■ James Paul Gee, *What Video Games Have to Teach Us About Learning and Literacy*, 2nd ed. (New York: Palgrave Macmillan, 2007), Chapter 2, 13–50. Posted in MyCourses.

■ Jane McGonigal, *Reality is Broken: Why Games Make Us Better and How They Can Change the World* (New York: Penguin, 2011), Introduction, 1–15. Posted in MyCourses.

Due by the start of class (11 AM ET):

- Complete your "Omeka" item in the administrative portal of the Hill Cumorah Legacy Project website.
    - Upload images of your artifact/primary source.
    - Provide Dublin Core Metadata, including a description of your artifact.

In class:

- Visit to the Magic Center with MAGIC Hub Coordinator Robert Mostyn.
- *Mission US*: https://www.mission-us.org/.
- *Never Alone*: http://neveralonegame.com/.
- *Play the Past*: http://www.playthepast.org/.

Week 9, March 6–March 13: Spring Break

Over spring break, play *Oregon Trail* on the Internet Archive and write a 750-word response about the experience. Additional instructions will be provided.

Our course's Imagine RIT proposal is due on March 11.

Week 10: Documentary Editing and Virtual History

Tuesday, March 15: Wikipedia, Online Encyclopedias, and Gender Bias

Read before class:

- Tamar Carroll and Lara Nicosia, "Wikipedia at 20: Why it often overlooks stories of women in history," *The Conversation*, Mar. 16, 2018, last modified Jan. 14, 2021, https://theconversation.com/wikipedia-at-20-why-it-often-overlooks-stories-of-women-in-history-92555. Approx. 3 pages.
- Katherine Maher, "Wikipedia is a mirror of the world's gender biases," Wikimedia Foundation, Oct. 18, 2018, https://wikimediafoundation.org/news/2018/10/18/wikipedia-mirror-world-gender-biases/. Approx. 3 pages.
- "What is TEI?" Univ. of Nebraska-Lincoln, https://cdrh.unl.edu/articles/basicguide/TEI. 3 pages.

Due by the start of class (11 AM ET): *Oregon Trail* response paper.

- Please submit your paper via MyCourses.

In class:

- Brief discussion about XML & TEI databases, using the Seward Project as an example (https://sewardproject.org/Databases). Then we'll segue into...
- Wikipedia Women's History Month Edit-a-Thon with Rebekah Walker.

Thursday, March 17: Scanning and Digitization

Update: No class on March 17. Tania Kleynhans's presentation was moved to Thursday, March 24.

Read before class:

■ Rosenzweig and Cohen, Digital History, "Becoming Digital," https://chnm.gmu.edu/digitalhistory/digitizing/. Approx. 28 pages.

■ Read **one** of the following:

- ■ National Archives, "FRMC White Paper: Digitization Cost Benefit Analysis," May 2019, https://www.archives.gov/files/frmc-digitization-cost-benefit-whitepaper.pdf. 8 pages.
- ■ National Archives, "Strategy for Digitizing Archival Materials for Public Access, 2015–2024," https://www.archives.gov/digitization/strategy.html. 6 pages.

■ Tania Kleynhans, MacKenzie L. Carr, and David W. Messenger, "Low-cost, user friendly multispectral imaging system for the recovery of damaged, faded or palimpsested historical documents," *Proceedings of SPIE* 11727, "Algorithms, Technologies, and Applications for Multispectral and Hyperspectral Imaging XXVII," 117270F (12 April 2021). 7 pages. Login with your RIT UID: https://doi.org/10.1117/12.2585629. Also on MyCourses.

In class:

■ Presentation by Tania Kleynhans from the RIT Center for Imaging Science (CIS) to discuss multispectral imaging.

Week 11: Digital Stories

Tuesday, March 22: Linear vs. Nonlinear Digital Storytelling

Read/watch before class:

■ Sadie Bergen, "Inside Ben Franklin's World: An Interview with Podcaster Liz Covart," *Perspectives on History*, Apr. 18, 2016, https://www.historians.org/publications-and-directories/perspectives-on-history/april-2016/inside-ben-franklins-world-an-interview-with-podcaster-liz-covart. Approx. 5 pages.

■ Paul Shoebridge and Michael Simons (The Goggles), "The Goggles," *Transom*, May 30, 2012, http://transom.org/?p=24352. Approx. 13 pages.

■ *Un(re)solved* web interactive experience by PBS (2021),: https://www.pbs.org/wgbh/frontline/unresolved/.

In class:

■ Twine storytelling workshop with Rebekah Walker.

■ Discussion of *Un(re)solved.*

For Reference:

- Additional storytelling apps:
    - ArcGIS Story Maps: https://storymaps.arcgis.com/.
    - Neatline: https://neatline.org/.
    - Scalar: https://scalar.me/anvc/scalar/.
    - Timeline JS from Knight Lab: https://timeline.knightlab.com/.
- Sample Projects:
    - Paul Shoebridge and Michael Simons (The Goggles), *Welcome to Pine Point*, National Film Board of Canada, https://pinepoint.nfb.ca/intro/#/info/project/64.
    - Scholastic's *Immigration: Stories of Yesterday and Today*: teacher.scholastic.com/activities/immigration/index.htm.

Thursday, March 24: No class. Work on your oral history interviews.
Update: Class after all. Tania Kleynhans's presentation.

Week 12: The Lifespan of Digital Projects

Tuesday, March 29: Preserving Digital Projects

Read before class:

- James Baker, "Preserving Your Research Data," *The Programming Historian* 3 (2014), https://doi.org/10.46430/phen0039. 9 pages.
- Quinn Dombrowski, "What Ever Happened to Project Bamboo?" *Literary and Linguistic Computing* 29, no. 3 (Sept. 2014): 326–39, https://doi.org/10.1093/llc/fqu026.

In class:

- Bamboo DiRT archived version: https://web.archive.org/web/20190928221355/http://dirtdirectory.org:80/.
- University of Victoria Endings Project, "Endings Principles for Digital Longevity": https://endings.uvic.ca/principles.html.
- *Slave Voyages 2.0*, "History of the Project": https://www.slavevoyages.org/about/about#history/1/en/. 2 pages.
- "The Socio-Technical Sustainability Roadmap," The Visual Media Workshop, University of Pittsburgh: https://sites.haa.pitt.edu/sustainabilityroadmap/.

Thursday, March 31: No class. Work on your oral history interviews.

Week 13: Transcribing Oral History

Tuesday, April 5: Introduction to Transcription Software

Due by the start of class (11 AM ET): Oral history recording.

- Please upload your WAV, M4A/AAC, or MP3 recording to RIT Google Drive.

In class:
- Introduction to transcribing AV recordings. What makes a quality transcript?
- Descript: https://www.descript.com/transcription.
- Express Scribe: https://www.nch.com.au/scribe/index.html.
- Otter.ai: https://otter.ai/pricing.
- RIT Guide to Captioning Panopto Videos: https://wiki.rit.edu/display/CourseVideo/Captioning+Course+Videos.
- Panopto Guide to Manual Captions: https://support.panopto.com/s/article/Manually-Caption-Your-Videos.
- Temi: https://www.temi.com/.

Thursday, April 7: No class. Work on your oral history transcripts.

Week 14: Group Work and Oral History Presentations

Tuesday, April 12: Transcription Practicum / Initial Website Review

Read before class:
- None. Work on your transcriptions.

In class:
- Look at the Omeka website and offer feedback.
- Work on your transcriptions in small groups.

Thursday, April 14: Presentations

Read before class:
- None. Work on your transcriptions.

Due by the start of class (11 AM ET): Oral history transcript.
- Please submit your transcript via MyCourses.

In class:
- First set of oral history project presentations.

Week 15: Oral History Presentations Continued

Tuesday, April 19: Presentations Continued
- Second set of oral history project presentations.
- Planning for Imagine RIT.

Thursday, April 21: Project Review and Course Conclusion
- In-class review of the Hill Cumorah Project website.
- Final discussion about digital history.

Saturday, April 23: Imagine RIT.

- We will present the work-in-progress version of the website to the public at Imagine RIT!

Weeks 16 and 17

Monday, April 25, 2022: Last day of RIT classes. We actually don't have class this week.
Tuesday, April 26, 2022: Reading Day.

Wednesday, April 27: Submit your "behind the scenes" paper via MyCourses by 5 PM.

April 27–29 and May 2–4, 2022: Final exam period.

Portions of this syllabus are adapted from prior digital history courses taught by Deborah Boyer (Villanova University, 2015), Dr. Michael Jarvis (University of Rochester, 2017), Dr. Camden Burd (RIT, 2019), and Dr. James Rankine (RIT, 2020). Some readings and concepts are derived from Natalie Baur's Library Juice Academy course "Ethics and Sustainability for Digital Curation."

I would like to thank the following people for their help with this course: Bentley Hutchings, Neil Pitts, Suzanne Stockman, and Brian Surprenant; Joshua Cotton and Monica Evans (Clark Atlanta University); Beth Slazak (Creative Education Foundation); Camden Burd (Eastern Illinois University); Konstantinos D. Karatzas (GIRES: Global Institute for Research, Education & Scholarship, Amsterdam, NL); Doug Boyd (University of Kentucky Louie B. Nunn Center for Oral History); Natalie Baur (Library Juice Academy); Robin Fay (Omeka); William Thomas and Patrick Jones (University of Nebraska–Lincoln); Jerry Argetsinger, Michael Brown, Katie Bush, Tamar Carroll, Monica Cormier, Cami Goldowitz, Chris Hedges, Ken Kindler, Tania Kleynhans, Patty Leight, Beth Midavaine, Robert Mostyn, Rebekah Walker, Leslie Weber, David Ziebarth, and the staff at IT Services (RIT); Jan Decker and the staff at the RIT Barnes & Noble bookstore; Gail Argetsinger (SUNY Brockport); Clara Auclair, Tom Devaney, Morris Eaves, James Rankine, Stephen Roessner, Josh Romphf, Emily Sherwood, Blair Tinker, and Lisa Wright (University of Rochester).

HIST 326 ORAL HISTORY PROJECT

Prof. Daniel Gorman Jr., RIT, Spring 2022

Working in pairs (or trios if necessary), you will conduct an oral history interview with a past participant in the Hill Cumorah Pageant. Your work will consist of three parts, which are outlined below—an initial list of ten questions for your interviewee, an audio recording of your interview, and a text transcript of your interview.

The materials you produce will go online at http://cumorahlegacy.omeka.net/, unless (a) you tell me via email by February 8, 2022, that you do not want your work to go online, and/or (b) your interviewee places restrictions on the interview materials.

Note: The students in each pair/trio will receive the same grade—unless it comes to my attention that one person did not contribute. In that case, the student who did the work will receive the grade, and the other student will receive an automatic failing grade on the project.

Part One: List of Questions

Due Thursday, February 17, 2022, 11 AM ET

Drawing on what you've learned from Matthew Bowman's book *The Mormon People*, Jerry Argetsinger and Brian Surprenant's presentations, and materials about the Hill Cumorah Pageant, you will create an initial **list of ten questions** for your interview subject. Be sure to write enough questions to fill a 25- to 40-minute interview.

Sample topics that you might discuss with your interviewee(s) include:

- Personal background: Hometown, education, profession, etc.
- Involvement in the Church of Jesus Christ of Latter-day Saints.
- How they became involved in the Hill Cumorah Pageant.
- Role(s) they performed in the Hill Cumorah Pageant. Examples: Acting, working behind-the-scenes, crowd management, refreshments, security/parking, missionary work, and/or advertising
- Memories of the Hill Cumorah Pageant.
- Favorite Book of Mormon story featured in the Pageant.
- The Pageant's cultural significance.
- The Pageant as a part of the Rochester area and Western New York's culture.
- Tourism and the Hill Cumorah Pageant.
- The end of the Pageant, including the Church's decision in 2018 to conclude its run and the COVID-19 pandemic.

Formatting Requirements:

- Your questions should be double-spaced and typed in 12-point font.
- Include the names of everyone in your group at the top of your document.
- Your document must include ten questions for your interviewee(s).

■ You do not need to include citations (Works Cited section, footnotes, or parenthetical citations) for this assignment.

Your questions are due at the start of class (11 AM ET) on Thursday, February 17. You will submit your questions via MyCourses. I will return your questions with comments. This assignment is worth 10% of your semester grade.

Note: Only one member of your group needs to submit the questions document on MyCourses. The "Group" feature in MyCourses will show the work and accompanying grade for all group members.

Part Two: Oral History Audio Recording
Due Tuesday, April 5, 2022, 11 AM ET

For Part Two of the project, you will meet with your interview subject either on Zoom or at an in-person location of your choice. You will interview your subject for a duration of 25 to 40 minutes and make an **audio recording** of the interview. **If you conduct the interview in person, be sure to record your interview in a quiet place to reduce background noise**.

It is fine if you do not discuss every question on your initial list. Oral history interviews tend to go in unexpected directions as the interviewee tells their story. It is better to follow up on an interesting comment than to stick to a rigid list of questions.

Assignment Requirements:

- The audio recording is between 25 and 40 minutes in length.
- **You must submit a signed consent form along with your recording.**
    - File Name Format: Include the last names of everyone in your group, the full name(s) of your interviewee(s), and the date. Example: Anderson_Brown_JohnColeConsentForm_03-02-2022.docx
- Please submit your interview as an audio file saved in MP3, M4A/AAC, or WAV format.
    - File Name Format: Include the last names of everyone in your group, the full name(s) of your interviewee(s), and the date. Example: Anderson_Brown_JohnColeInterview_03-02-2022.mp3
- If you record your interview with Zoom, the app will automatically create a video file and an MP3 audio file. You do not need to submit the video file.
- You will submit your interview audio recording AND the consent form to Google Drive.

Your recording is due at the start of class (11 AM ET) on Tuesday, April 5. This assignment is worth 15% of your semester grade.

Update, 3/13/2022: Students must respond to their group's introductory email thread (consisting of interviewers, interviewees, and Prof. Gorman) by 11:59 PM on Thursday, March 17. This way, there will be time for Prof. Gorman and community contact Bentley Hutchings to follow up with interviewees before the assignment due date. Failure to respond to introductory emails by the end of the day on 3/17 will result in five points being deducted from each group's final audio recording grade.

Part Three: Oral History Transcript
Due Thursday, April 14, 2022, 11 AM ET

For Part Three, you will produce a text **transcript** of your interview. This transcript will accompany your audio recording on the Hill Cumorah Legacy Project website. By creating a transcript, you will make your transcript **searchable** and **accessible to website visitors of all abilities**.

You must use one of the following apps (or another equivalent app) to produce an initial transcript:

- Descript: https://www.descript.com/transcription.
- Express Scribe: https://www.nch.com.au/scribe/index.html.
- Otter.ai: https://otter.ai/pricing.
- RIT Guide to Captioning Panopto Videos: https://wiki.rit.edu/display/CourseVideo/Captioning+Course+Videos.
- Panopto Guide to Manual Captions: https://support.panopto.com/s/article/Manually-Caption-Your-Videos.
- Temi: https://www.temi.com/.

Assignment Requirements:

- Once you have produced your initial transcript in a transcription app, copy the text into a word processing app.
- File Name Format: Include the last names of everyone in your group, the full name(s) of your interviewee(s), and the date.
  - Example: Anderson_Brown_JohnColeTranscript_03-02-2022.docx
- Your transcript should be double-spaced and typed in 12-point font.
- At the start of the transcript document, include a title for your interview with the interviewee's name and the date of recording.
- Below the title, include the names of everyone in your group and the name of the transcription app you used.
- Identify all speakers throughout the transcript with their full names.
- Add timestamps in five-minute increments (00:00, 05:00, etc.) throughout the transcript.
- Proofread your transcript for grammar errors.
- Remove filler words like "like," "um," and "uh" from the transcript.
- Add any relevant hyperlinks to the transcript.
- After the text of your transcript, provide Dublin Core Metadata categories (listed below) about your interview.

Your final transcript is due at the start of class (11 AM ET) on Thursday, April 14. You will submit your transcript and Dublin Core information as a single .docx file via MyCourses. This assignment is worth 10% of your semester grade.

Note: Only one member of your group needs to submit the transcript document on MyCourses. The "Group" feature in MyCourses will show the work and accompanying grade for all group members.

Dublin Core Metadata Categories for Your Oral History Interview

Title: "A name given to the resource."

■ A title for your interview with the interviewee's name and the date of recording.

Subject: "The topic of the resource."

■ Aside from "Hill Cumorah Project," you could list any topics that came up repeatedly during the interview.

Description: "An account of the resource."

■ For the Hill Cumorah Legacy Project, this will be a paragraph that is at least 100 words in length, introducing your interviewee and summarizing the content of the interview.

Creator: "An entity primarily responsible for making the resource."

■ The "Creator" category should include the interviewee's or interviewees' name(s) as well as the interviewers' names.

Source: "A related resource from which the described resource is derived."

■ You can simply write "Hill Cumorah Legacy Project" here.

Date: "A point or period of time associated with an event in the lifecycle of the resource."

■ This is the date on which you conducted your interview.

Contributor: "An entity responsible for making contributions to the resource."

■ The names of your group members go here.

Rights: "Information about rights held in and over the resource."

■ If the interviewee places no restrictions on the interview, then you will write: "Produced under an oral history collaborative deed of gift agreement with no restrictions and nonexclusive license."

■ If the interviewee places restrictions on the interview, then you will write: "Produced under an oral history collaborative deed of gift agreement with restrictions and nonexclusive license."

Format: "The file format, physical medium, or dimensions of the resource."

■ List the file format (MP3, M4A/AAC, or WAV) in which you recorded your interview.

Language: A language of the resource.

■ This will probably be English unless another language is used during part of the interview.

Identifier: "An unambiguous reference to the resource within a given context."

■ This will be the file name(s) of the photo(s) of your object that you upload.

Source Note: The definitions in quotation marks for each metadata element are taken from: DCMI Usage Board, "Dublin Core™ Metadata Element Set, Version 1.1: Reference Description," Dublin Core Metadata Innovation, last modified June 14, 2012. https://www.dublincore.org/specifications/dublin-core/dces/.

ROC ARTIFACT

Moses Shongo's Wallpaper

Cynthia Van Ness

When the Hotel Seneca opened at the intersection of Main and Clinton in downtown Rochester in September 1908, it had 10 stories; 350 rooms; Otis elevators; and a bathtub, shower, and long-distance telephone in every room.[1] It also had custom wallpaper designed by Moses Shongo (ca. 1860–1925), which was manufactured by the M.H. Birge & Sons wallcovering company of Buffalo, New York. The hotel architectural firm was Esenwein and Johnson, also of Buffalo.[2] The hotel's inaugural event was hosting the convention of the New York State Democratic Party.[3]

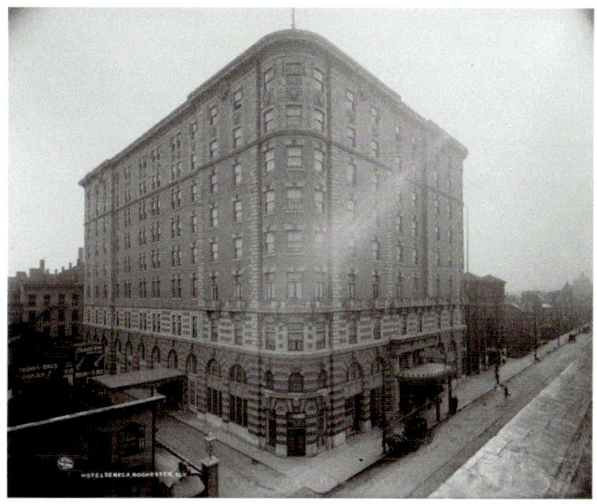

Hotel Seneca. *Detroit Publishing Company (ca. 1910),* Hotel Seneca, Rochester, NY, *photograph, Washington, DC: Library of Congress, accessed February 23, 2024, https://www.loc.gov/item/2016810434/.*

Moses Shongo (*Ho non da a suh,* "Keeper of the hills"[4]) was a member of the Seneca Nation Wolf Clan and lived on the Cattaraugus reservation, 100 miles southwest of Rochester. He was an accomplished cornet player and band leader, a composer, a lecturer, and a teacher at several Indian schools, and he held various roles on the reservation. During the Spanish American war, Shongo served with the 10th US Cavalry, a segregated regiment.[5] In 1901, he performed with the Carlisle Indian Band at Buffalo's Pan-American Exposition. He was a traditional medicine man but also a convert to Christianity.

From ca. 1903 until his death in 1925, Shongo worked at the Buffalo Historical Society (now The Buffalo History Museum),

Cynthia Van Ness began her library career as a page at the Rochester Public Library. She holds an MS in library science from the University at Buffalo and has served as the director of Library and Archives at The Buffalo History Museum since 2007. She is the author of *Victorian Buffalo: Images from the Buffalo and Erie County Public Library* (1999) and *Quotable Buffalo* (2011). In her own time, she is the webmaster of BuffaloResearch.com, founded in 1993, a portal for researching Buffalo ancestors and architecture and Buffalo's oldest surviving website. She can be contacted at AskBuffaloResearch@gmail.com.

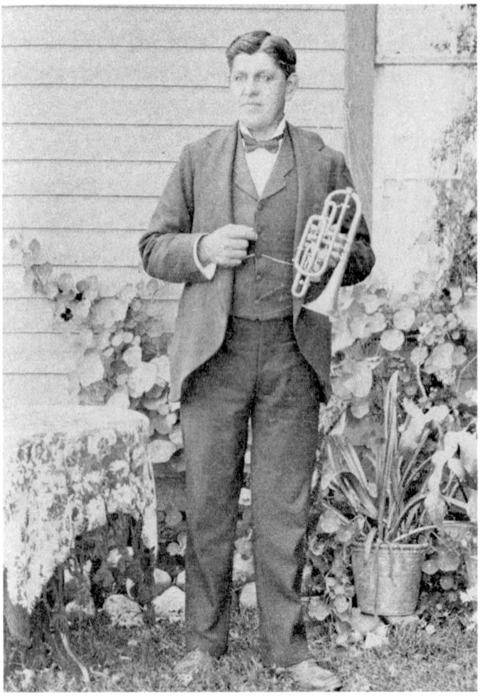

Portrait of Moses Shongo. *Edward Hale Brush,* Iroquois Past and Present, *1900. E-book, Buffalo, NY: Baker, Jones and Company, accessed February 18, 2024, https://www.loc.gov/item/07006948/.*

starting as a janitor and attaining, around 1912,[6] the position of curator. This author has been unable to identify any other Native Americans working in a curatorial capacity at that time, making him the first- or earliest-known museum curator of Native descent in the United States.

Shongo's wallpaper design is known to us today only via this page, perhaps pulled out of an unidentified M.H. Birge company or Hotel Seneca publication and found in the vertical files of the Research Library at The Buffalo History Museum. It is now online at Archive.org.[7]

Handwritten notes in pencil, probably by Shongo, read, "Nun-Do-Wak-O-Noh means people of the great hill. Tsonontouans as near as the French would pronounce it. Dots and dash lines are wampum belts. Star the capitol of Five Nations. Five feathers pointing to the star are the five nations. Lacrosse stick within it work for original Indian game. Tanned animal skin pictures with different animals and birds for clans."

The printed caption indicates that Shongo's wallpaper was used in halls and corridors at the Hotel Seneca. No photographs of the wallpaper in situ are known to exist. Later renamed the Manger Hotel, the Seneca was demolished in 1969 and is presently the site of the Windstream (Paetec) building.

How Shongo came to design this wallpaper is unknown. It is likely that either August C. Esenwein (1855–1926) and James A. Johnson (1865–1939), the hotel's architects, or hotel co-owner H. M. (Henry Montgomery) Gerrans (1853–1939),[8] all of Buffalo, played a part. Gerrans also owned the Hotel Iroquois in Buffalo, which opened in 1889 and may have inspired the Hotel Seneca's name and theme. All three men would have been well acquainted with Birge company wallpapers. In turn, Birge may have reached out to Shongo, who by this time was regularly performing and lecturing in Buffalo.

The M.H. Birge company, founded in Buffalo by Martin Howland Birge (1806–1900), began manufacturing wallpaper in 1834 and developed an international reputation for excellent craftsmanship and engagement with the major artistic movements of the twentieth century, most notably Arts and Crafts, Art Deco, and Art Nouveau.[9] Another company specialty was colonial reproduction wallpapers. The company ceased operations in 1982. The Victoria and Albert Museum in London maintains a collection of Birge wallcoverings.[10]

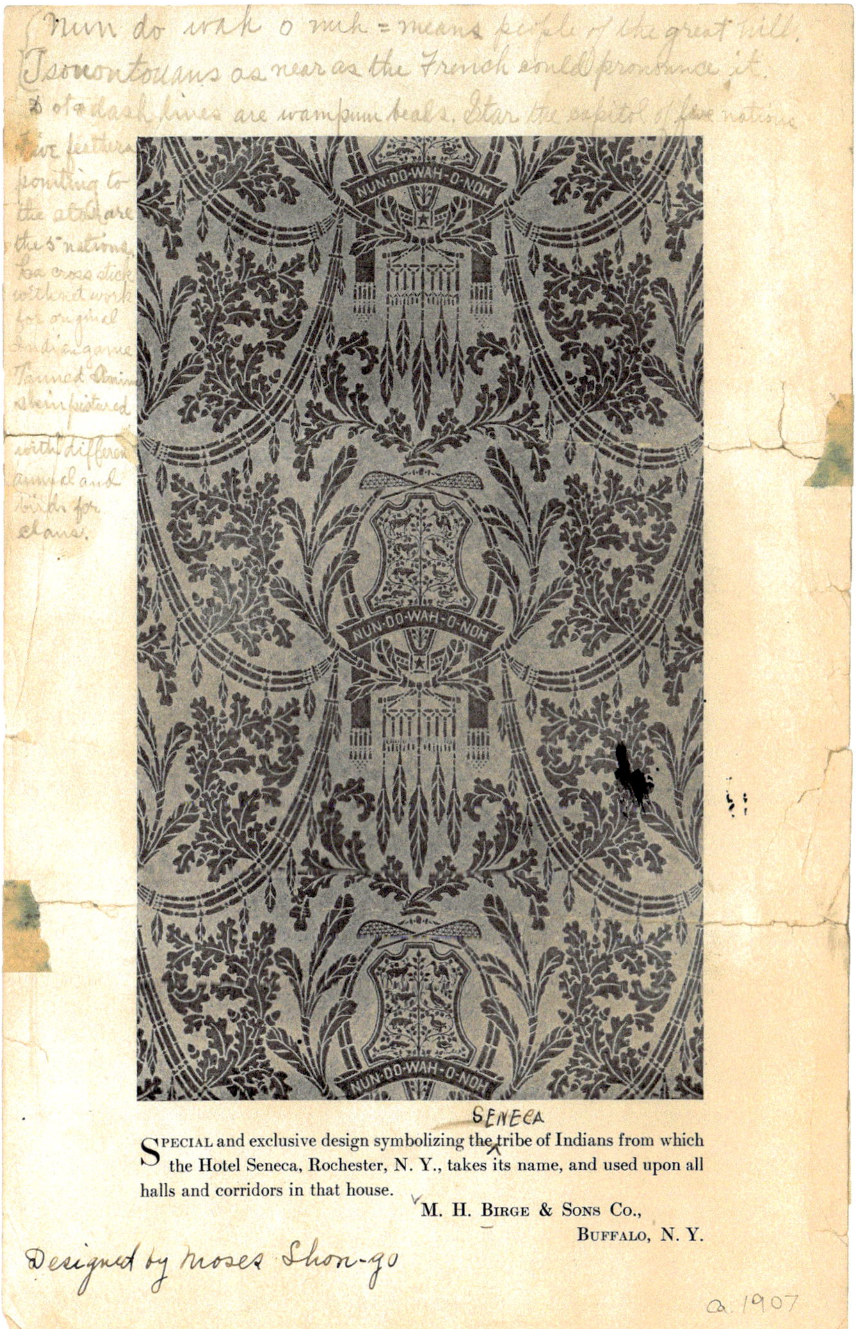

Shongo's wallpaper. *The Buffalo History Museum, "Moses Shongo's Wallpaper," 2024.*

Around 1903, the Buffalo Historical Society engraved this motto by Shongo in marble over a prominent doorway, in Seneca and English, where visitors can still see it today:

NEH-KO, GAH-GIS-DAH-YEN-DUK

OTHER COUNCIL FIRES WERE HERE BEFORE OURS.

While the Hotel Seneca did exploit Haudenosaunee (Six Nations) themes for commercial gain, it also enabled a Seneca Indian to direct one of its design choices, a small but inclusive and pioneering gesture in 1908. ■

1 "Box Convention: Preparations About Completed for Summer Meeting to Be Held at Rochester, N.Y.," 1910. *The Packages* 13 (7): 41, accessed February 18, 2024, https://books.google.com/books?id=IwVZAAAAYAAJ&pg=RA6-PA41&dq=%22Hotel+Seneca%22+Rochester&hl=en&newbks=1&newbks_redir=0&sa=X&ved=2ahUKEwjfwfednrWEAxUQC3kGHWTDBx0Q6AF6BAgLEAI#v=onepage&q=%22Hotel%20Seneca%22%20Rochester&f=false.

2 "New Yorkers Will Build Hotel Seneca," *Buffalo Times*, March 24, 1907.

3 "Democrats Will Name State Ticket Today: Candidates Will Be Choices of the People," *Buffalo Courier*, September 16, 1908.

4 Mabel Powers, *Stories the Iroquois Tell Their Children*, 1917. E-book, New York: American Book Company, accessed February 18, 2024, https://www.gutenberg.org/files/22096/22096-h/22096-h.htm.

5 "Kin, Friends of Moses Shongo, Late Cattaraugus Indian, Will Serve Meal for Departed Spirit," *Buffalo Courier*, September 27, 1925.

6 Buffalo Historical Society, 1926, "Necrology: Buffalonians More or Less Prominent Who Died During the Year 1925," *Reports of the President and Secretary Submitted at the Annual Meeting, January 12, 1926*, 64 (January): 87, accessed February 20, 2024, https://babel.hathitrust.org/cgi/pt?id=uc1.$b728264&seq=195.

7 The Buffalo History Museum, 2024, "Moses Shongo's Wallpaper," *Vertical File: Manufacturers—Birge*, Archive.Org, January 13, 2024, accessed February 18, 2024, https://archive.org/details/shongo-moses-wallpaper. No standalone collection of Shongo's papers survive, though a few articles by him are in Folder 15 of the Museum's *Indian Collection* (Mss. B00-2), a manuscript collection assembled from multiple sources after his death.

8 "Hotel Seneca Is Ready for Furnishings," *Buffalo Sunday Morning News*, August 16, 1908, p. 7.

9 Bonnie Urich, "The M.H. Birge & Sons Company: A Design Wonderland in Buffalo," *Western New York Heritage* 14 (3), 2011, accessed February 18, 2024, https://www.wnyheritage.org/issue/fall_2011/index.html.

10 Victoria and Albert Museum, "Wallpaper: Early 29th Century," n.d., V&A, accessed February 18, 2024, https://collections.vam.ac.uk/item/O198699/wallpaper-m-h-birge/.